GERRY

by
MARY MURTON
with
MARY KERR

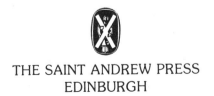

THE SAINT ANDREW PRESS
EDINBURGH

First published in 1982 by
THE SAINT ANDREW PRESS
121 George Street, Edinburgh EH2 4YN

Copyright © Mary Murton, 1982

ISBN 0 7152 0496 3

Printed in Hong Kong by Permanent Typesetting & Printing Co., Ltd.

GERRY

CONTENTS

AUTHOR'S PREFACE

This book has been very difficult to write. In fact, I wrote it so badly that, had it not been for the work of Mary Kerr, who edited it, there would not have been a book called *Gerry* published. Mary and I met through the publishing company, and I now know her as a friend whose devoted work on this book has made it almost as much hers as mine. Some of the photographs in the book were taken by her husband Scott.

I would never have written Gerry's story at all had it not been for Eric Fisher. He told me to 'tell people about Gerry'. He felt that this story might help other people to face terminal illness in a child. So, in the hope that it might help someone, somewhere, I set out to write it all down. My first efforts were 'properly' typed out by another friend, Irene Newell, to whom go more thanks, as no publisher would have wanted to read my first typescript!

My deepest gratitude goes to God Himself who, through Jesus Christ, has been at the centre of my life and who has given me the strength to face everything life has had in store for me. I know that my Redeemer liveth, and that He will be with me always, 'to the end of the age'. Thanks to Gerry, I also know that 'It's going to be ever so exciting when I die, much nicer than here.'

If anyone reading this little book is helped at all, please give all the thanks and the glory to God.

Mary Murton

May, 1981   Inverchapel Farm

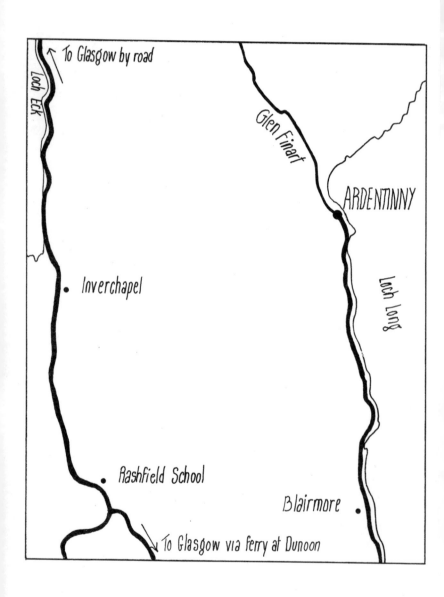

1. A DIFFERENT LIFE

'I'm going to get better, Jesus told me I would.'

So said Gerry when he opened his eyes after receiving two pints of blood in hospital. The year was 1969. He was four-and-a-half years old, and the doctor had just diagnosed leukemia.

'He may live for six weeks,' the doctor had said, 'he may even live for two years, but right now he is a very sick child.'

Then began a new and different life for us. We had all the anxiety of Gerry's illness, plus moving into the hotel we had bought that very week. My husband Trevor and I, together with our three sons, Paul, Bram and Gerry, had just moved to Ardentinny in the west of Scotland from Bridge of Weir in Renfrewshire. It was our first venture into the hotel business and, naturally, we were anxious that all would go well.

When the news of Gerry's illness sank in, we realised that we were suddenly 'different'. We knew our child would die. We all know that someday we are going to die, but to us death became very real. Perhaps it is true that ignorance is bliss.

I knew that our two older boys could easily be killed by a car, or die in some other way before Gerry, but it still made Gerry special in that, consciously or not, we cherished every moment of his life from then on. It also made me cherish Paul and Bram that bit more. Forgetfulness of our own mortality makes us take even our nearest and dearest ones for granted.

Three weeks later I took Gerry home from the hospital against the doctor's wishes. He was much better, and he screamed every night when I had to leave him in the big, old-fashioned hospital in Glasgow. He was not used to the Glaswegian accents of the staff, and their kindly enquiries, 'Will ye hae a piece an' jam, sonny?' were totally incomprehensible to him and only made him feel more homesick for his 'English' mum and family.

Despite the official censure of my action in taking Gerry away from the hospital, one young Sister quietly told me she would have done the same thing if he were her child. I felt that he might as well die at home, happy, as die in hospital where he was so miserable.

Gerry was an attractive child, with blue eyes and the brightest golden hair which just curled round his ears. Big for his age, and quite intelligent, he brightened up as soon as I told him he was going home. I was given a card to take him to the clinic the following week, and off we went to our new home. Gerry had been bitterly disappointed not to have been with us when we had moved to the hotel in Ardentinny three weeks previously. It was a seventy-mile car journey from the hospital in Glasgow, but we were able to cut down the mileage appreciably by using the car ferry from Gourock to Dunoon and then driving round the coast to Ardentinny.

To help out with visiting Gerry while he was in hospital, my mother, who lives with us, and my mother-in-law had stayed with friends who lived near Glasgow. They were thus able to be at the hospital most of each day with their beloved grandson. Neither of them knew that Gerry had leukemia. We told them he was very ill with acute anaemia. Only a few friends were told of the seriousness of the situation, as we did not want Gerry to find out that he was likely to die very soon, and in any case he was spoiled enough by his grandmothers as it was.

Home! What a wonderful place that is — even if it is a new home. If your heart is there, then it is the best place in the world. We were especially blessed in our new situation. Ardentinny is a beautiful, peaceful little village in the county of Argyll. It stands on the shore of Loch Long, a sea loch, and is bordered by hills and forest. It was ideal for Gerry.

Within a week he had made such a remarkable recovery that, when I took him to the clinic in Glasgow the following Thursday, the doctor was visibly impressed.

I constantly prayed that God would not let Gerry suffer. I could let him go to God, but I could not bear to see him in pain or unhappy. He had had pain in his legs before he went into hospital, and that had been unbearable. After that, the only pain was that of the bone marrow tests and spinal injections. His unhappiness at being parted from me while he was in hospital had been overwhelming, for we had rarely been apart. The other boys had had the opportunity of going to stay with their grandparents when we lived in England, but we had moved to Scotland when Gerry was only two years old.

Because of Gerry's treatment, we began a routine of weekly visits to the clinic in Glasgow, made more difficult because I had to get home in time to cook dinner for our guests which was served at 7.30 p.m. This meant that my mother, who had once thought she had retired, had to deal with the lunches and run the bar, as well as make the preparations for dinner. Trevor was still working as a civil engineer agent at this time, coming home at the weekends to take care of the bar. We never thought my mother would end up being the 'barmaid', but it turned out that she had to be. Actually, she was very popular, and listened patiently to people's troubles and tales.

The weeks went by quickly, and I continued to take Gerry to the clinic every Thursday. Then, one week, the doctor announced that there had been a breakthrough in the treatment of leukemia in children. Would we let Gerry have intensive chemotherapy for six weeks? What a difficult question! There was Gerry, so well and happy; should we allow him to go into hospital to have this treatment? After a great deal of thought and discussion, and some prayer on my part, we decided that we had better let him have the treatment. If only I had listened to the voice within me which said 'No', but in those days I was far too busy to take any notice of 'the still small voice'.

I wrote to my mother-in-law and told her what was really wrong with Gerry. There was still no need to tell my mother. I also asked 'Nan Ted', as she was known, if she would come up to Scotland for six weeks to do the hospital visiting. That six weeks became thirteen weeks, during which time Gerry was to be in hospital for periods of six days with a drip attached to his ankle or wrist. If his blood count was too low for the next drip, he would come home for a day or two before going back into hospital. He spent his fifth birthday in hospital, but was allowed out for a day in the country as he was off the drip. In fact, we went to a smart hotel, and he had a super birthday lunch — a thing he ever after wanted to repeat!

For Gerry's birthday we bought him a pony, a small white Welsh pony called Barney. We thought his legs might always be weak and riding on Barney was a marvellous way to get Gerry into the fresh air. It was on a 'pony walk' in the forest behind Ardentinny that I tried to explain to Gerry, then just five years old, that he should try to take in all the beauty of the mountains and forest and scenery, all God's creation, and fill himself with it in order to get strong and well.

He looked at me and said, 'Don't be silly, Mum, I can't get the mountains in my tummy.' Then he gave a grin, and said in that strange grown-up way he had, 'You mean I should absorb it all.'

I felt silly, I don't believe in using baby talk to any child, but I really didn't think he would have understood the word 'absorb'.

The remarkable thing about the thirteen weeks of chemotherapy treatment was that, in answer to everyone's prayers, Gerry was not at all miserable. Contrary to his unahppy state during his first stay in hospital, he was the life and soul of the ward. He was usually the centre of attraction: drawing pictures of birds for adoring nurses, or talking about microscopes to young doctors.

Every day his grandmother, 'Nan Ted', spent the day with him. I was only able to go to the hospital once a week. On that day my mother and mother-in-law were left at the hotel. With the help of the staff they coped, and had the dinner ready for me to dish up when I got home, often on the dot of 7.30. On hospital visits Gerry would get very cross with me for, not being used to the inactivity of the ward, I would sometimes fall asleep across his bed. One evening I felt sleepy driving home and had to pull off the road. I promptly fell asleep in the car. I think I was more exhausted at that time than I cared to admit.

At the end of thirteen weeks Gerry came home for good. We had a belated birthday party for him which was combined with Paul's twelfth birthday. To Gerry's delight, Dougal himself from the television programme 'The Magic Roundabout' came to the party. ('Dougal' was the father of Emma and Sophie, two friends the boys had made in the village.) It was a great party — with a cake looking like Dougal, as well as the traditional cake with candles on it. Gerry had received two cakes for his birthday in hospital, one from me and one kindly made by the hospital staff, but home was the place for a proper birthday party.

2. HOME, SWEET HOME

One of our first concerns in the new hotel venture was to get staff. Also, I was concerned to have someone to help me look after Gerry. I knew I would be very busy just at the time he should be having his bath and going to bed.

Just the right person turned up — a schoolgirl whom we had known in our previous home town of Bridge of Weir. She often used to walk our labrador dog, Nick. Gerry was very fond of Anne, and she of him. She came to work for us that first Easter when we opened the hotel, and came regularly during the school holidays after that. On her first Saturday night, Anne helped out with waiting at table. She was quite inexperienced but she was such a happy girl that she was very popular and received lots of tips. She had her share of embarrassing incidents though — like the time she dropped a whole dish of peas on the dining room floor!

The mainstay of our staff was a local lady, Mrs Ewing, who had worked, on and off, at the hotel since she first came to Ardentinny as a girl. Her pride and joy was the dining room, which was beautifully kept. A grandmother herself, she was very patient with Gerry. He went through a phase of hiding under the tablecloths and then jumping out to startle the guests. Mrs Ewing would shout, 'You young rascal', and chase him out of the room in fun. The guests seemed to enjoy all these antics, and Gerry got very spoilt by them.

They seemed to enjoy the music and laughter that emanated from the kitchen too. Two of our student helpers were keen on the proms, as was I. We used to have the radio on in the kitchen and we often found ourselves

6

dancing through into the dining room with trays of food and having hurriedly to compose ourselves.

Gerry made friends with an American couple who visited for a weekend. It turned out that the man's great-grandfather had once owned the hotel. They took him out with them so he could show them round the village. At breakfast he showed them how to fillet their kippers so that they could be eaten with the minimum of bones. At five years old he loved kippers, and was already an expert at dissecting them. The couple took a great liking to Gerry, though I don't know what they thought of his habit of putting plastic spiders in tea cups and stuffed mice on the cheese board!

During the years we had the hotel lots of amusing incidents took place. On one memorable occasion we had a small fire in the kitchen. Flames were seen licking up from the wires at the back of the cooker. Without even stopping to think, I grabbed the fire extinguisher and pointed it at the flames. It contained powder, not foam, and soon everything in the kitchen, including all the staff, was covered with a fine white layer. If it had not been for the quick thinking of my mother-in-law, all the guests' food for the evening would have been ruined. She quickly threw a tablecloth over the plates of food in the nick of time.

Although the fire was soon out, I couldn't turn the fire extinguisher off. Whichever way I turned, trying to stop it, a thick layer of powder was deposited. Finally, with the help of a guest, I did manage to turn it off. By then we were all covered with white powder and looked as though we had suddenly gone grey with shock. What a mess we had to clear up that day!

As for Gerry, he thrived on all the fun and I am sure it was in part due to the atmosphere in our home that he kept so well. Most mornings, after Paul and Bram had gone off on the school bus and before I started making breakfast for the guests, I would take Gerry out on Barney the pony. Those early morning rides, as well as being good for Gerry, ensured my daily dose of fresh air, for I found the hotel to be very much an indoor job. It was also a great opportunity to be alone with Gerry and we both enjoyed the special times we spent together.

Life was very busy that first summer, so when Trevor suggested a short break I was delighted. Only once before had we all been on holiday together, and that had been for a week in a caravan in Sutherland. We decided on the island of Mull, off the west coast of Scotland, and booked into a hotel for a long weekend.

Leaving my mother and a friend in charge of our hotel, we set off on a fine sunny day with excitement running high. The view from the ferry as we crossed to the island was breathtaking. Though I have since made that journey many times, I still have to stay on deck the entire time so as not to miss anything. To the east the mountains of Glencoe tower majestically and Ben Cruachan stands aloof and grand beyond the picturesque fishing port of Oban. That morning the sea sparkled in the sunlight and the screaming gulls swooped and dived around the ferry hoping for scraps from the entranced passengers.

We picnicked just off the road after we landed. Gerry, always interested in birds and wildlife in general, was thrilled to see a buzzard on a fence. In fact, we saw so many buzzards, and herons too, that the novelty soon wore off. All three boys were full of beans that day and they had a good tumble and roll on the grassy bank we had chosen for our picnic.

We decided to make our way almost immediately to the hotel we had booked into. When we arrived we found that the bed in the room we had been given was a 'Scottish' double bed — too short for Trevor's 6 feet 4 inches. We were given another room without too much fuss, but that was just the first of a number of incidents which were to mar our holiday.

I was looking forward to a nice meal which I hadn't had to prepare, and, since it was our wedding anniversary, Trevor had planned to order a bottle of wine. When we went down to dinner, however, we found that not only was there no choice offered, but that the food was very poorly cooked and presented. Apparently a film was being made locally and the hotel proprietors, assured of their bookings, did not seem to care whether their guests were happy or not. Needless to say, we did not waste our money on the wine!

The next morning Paul discovered that his bedspread, which looked perfectly clean, smelt revolting. It seemed that a previous guest had been sick on it and it had not been properly washed. He was very upset needless to say. The biggest shock of all, though, was the bill when we came to leave. We found that we had been charged far more than we charged at our own hotel, despite the poor food and service and the fact that all three boys shared a room.

Despite the disappointments, though, we had an enjoyable break and did lots of exploring. Mull has dramatic scenery, and I was enthralled by the apparent vastness of the place. Glimpses of islands whenever we saw the sea reminded us of the fact that we were also on an island, although we didn't feel as if we were. The cliffs at Calgary towered above us, and we saw a curious seal who stared at us with huge brown eyes. Here the sea really was 'the ocean', with huge breakers which rolled in along the wide sandy beaches.

The skeleton of an old boat on the marshy shores of Loch Scridain drew Trevor like a magnet. He was a sailor at heart, and couldn't resist anything that looked even vaguely like a boat. He thought that the old hulk would be worth burning to get the wealth of copper nails out of her, for that was all the weather-beaten bones held that were of any value. The boys followed their dad faithfully, imitating his interest as boys always do.

I saw a sign announcing 'Iona Ferry'.

'Let's go,' I said, but Trevor said we had no time for a visit just then.

Little did I realise that I would later spend many happy

days on that holy isle and form friendships there which I believe will last for all eternity.

3. SPECIAL TREATMENT

That year, as an addition to his intensive treatment, Gerry was to be one of the first three children in Glasgow to have a new series of vaccinations against leukemia. They were very painful, and he had to endure a year of them in his arms and thighs.

Despite the treatment, the year was a happy one. Gerry went from strength to strength and no one could possibly have guessed that he had leukemia, least of all his adoring grandmother. For one thing, he started school. Gerry had been unable to attend the village school whilst he had been in and out of hospital, so a good friend had been coming in each evening for an hour after teaching in Dunoon. She taught Gerry a great deal, lessons which stood him in good stead for the rest of his school life. In fact, he became quite big-headed when he eventually started school because he was so far ahead of the other children.

Time at Ardentinny school was quite idyllic compared to most people's schooldays. The children had only to run down the street, and the little school was situated right by the side of the loch. It was a tiny, one-teacher school with only about fifteen pupils. There began a great friendship of the 'David and Jonathan' variety. Gerry met Eddie, a year older than himself, and they became inseparable. Gerry's passion for birds and wildlife grew, and the two boys would roam in the forest or along the shore for hours.

One Sunday both were missing at lunchtime. A search was made but there was no sign of either of them and no one had seen them for hours. The sea was rough and angry and waves were even crashing against the rocks in our

11

garden. I searched along the shore, praying that they had not been drowned. At about three o'clock in the afternoon they were found, two miles up the glen, playing happily in a big sand hole at the side of the road. Boys! I thanked God for their safety and the fact that Gerry was able to be a normal boy, and do normal things like getting lost.

Exactly a year to the day after Gerry began having the vaccinations, it was found that he had had too many. As a result a small tumour had appeared in a most embarrassing place. Gerry had to have radiotherapy for a few weeks which, though not painful, was embarrassing for him. He had to take several courses of drugs as well and at that time he had to take so many tablets that he was awarded a special 'Blue Peter' prize for being a 'champion tablet taker'. 'Blue Peter' was the boys' favourite television programme in those days.

It was during this period of his life that Gerry seemed to become particularly close to God. He had always believed in God, but now his faith was becoming much stronger. One night he said to me, 'It's going to be ever so exciting when I die — much nicer than here!' He often spoke as if he had a knowledge of the next life which he took for granted.

Gerry always loved to hear stories from the Bible, particularly stories of the nativity and speculations as to what Jesus did when He was a little boy. Sadly, the older boys had grown away from such things. Strangely, Gerry also loved to hear about the crucifixion and resurrection — perhaps because he knew how much 'nicer' it was going to be after this life is finished for everyone who loves God.

One day we had to go to hospital by public transport — a thing we rarely did because it took longer and was uncomfortable for Gerry if he had to have an injection. On that day, as usual, I had a book to read to Gerry, but as we took the ferry across the River Clyde we were too busy sightseeing to need a story. It was quite an event for us to go on a train, and we went in the front coach so that Gerry could be near the driver. The usual assortment of people, all minding their own business, were on the train: some American sailors from the submarine base in the nearby Holy Loch; young women with children; old women watching the little ones.

To my complete surprise, instead of coming to me and asking me to read him a story, Gerry came up and said in a loud voice, 'Mum, tell me the story of Jesus!'

I was embarrassed — it seemed rather odd to start telling that story in a crowded train.

'Go on, you know how it starts,' Gerry ordered.

And so it was that I told the story of Jesus, in a loud voice, in a railway carriage quite full of people. Once I got started I forgot my embarrassment and saw only the blue eyes of Gerry looking into mine. I knew then what Jesus meant when He said that we should become 'like little children'.

Gerry liked to come to church with me on Sundays and we usually went to the communion service at Holy Trinity Episcopal Church in Dunoon. I was quite friendly with our local Church of Scotland minister in Ardentinny, but, being an Anglican, I preferred to travel the twelve miles to a church where the service was more familiar.

One Sunday Gerry was kneeling beside me at the altar rail. I had just taken communion and the rector moved on to Gerry and, as usual, placed his hands on the little head to bless him. I felt a strange movement in the air, as though a rug were being shaken beside me. I peeped through my fingers, but all was normal — the rector was not shaking his robe or anything like that.

I continued to think about the strange experience after the service but, unlike my usual self, I did not mention it to anyone at first. Then on the following Tuesday, when I was on the way to the hospital with Gerry, I spoke about the incident.

'You know on Sunday, when the rector put his hands on your head . . .'

'Yes.'

'Well, what did he do?'

'Oh, Mummy, it was lovely,' said Gerry enthusiastically. 'I felt all happy and nice, like on Christmas morning when you wake up and know there are presents.'

A few days later I told the rector about it. He said he had not felt anything, and seemed to think it must have been Gerry's and my imagination. However, some time later I began to read about, and hear about, people having similar experiences. In any case, how could a six-year-old imagine that sort of experience?

Months later, when Gerry, Bram and I were talking about knowing God, Gerry said, 'I know what heaven is like — it's like the lovely feeling of lightness and brightness I felt through my hair that time in church.'

Bram, then nine, felt he was missing out.

'It's not fair, you and Mum know God, and I don't!' he said to Gerry.

But it was just that Gerry had experienced so much in such a short time. He had been close to death, and I believe that through that he had become close to God. I was always saddened at the hospital to see little children completely engrossed in football teams or pop stars. Didn't their mothers tell them anything that mattered? I feel very strongly that a sick child, and certainly a dying one, should be surrounded by beauty, be filled with heavenly things.

I thought I knew God at that time, too. But I was to get to know Him so much better through the trials, and heartaches our family would have to face in the years to come. Born again by the Spirit of God in Chester Cathedral at eighteen years of age, I had tried to serve Him faithfully since then. But I had so much more to learn of the wonderful grace of God and of His complete faithfulness — and Gerry, a small boy of six, was helping to teach me.

4. EVERYDAY LIFE

A regular routine of fortnightly visits to the clinic in Glasgow continued to be our way of life. Gerry carried on taking his tablets and lived a very happy, active life.

Gerry was always very bright for his age and, as he grew older, he developed many skills and interests. From an early age he had his future mapped out. As a small boy he had made a special prayer for guidance.

'Almighty God, king of all the universe,' he had prayed, 'tell me what to do when I grow up.'

He believed that God wanted him to become a doctor. He was fascinated with medical diagrams, and had a 'Visible Man', one of those models which come apart and show all the organs of the human body. When he was about seven or eight he compiled a book, which I still have, containing drawings of different parts of the body. I showed it to one of the hospital doctors who thought it quite remarkable for one so young. Some of the entries are interesting. A drawing of the brain bears the caption 'Your bran is mad of meni nerves', and goes on to inform the reader, 'Wen you Get Goos pipols it is your nerves aer pooling the hers on your Body tite.' Spelling never was Gerry's strong point!

Among Gerry's pets were two goldfish. One day we found one of the fish dead. We suspected that it was because they had been put into a newly-cemented pond, and quickly rescued the second one. Gerry decided that he should dissect the dead fish to see why it had died.

'I don't really like doing it, Mum,' he said, 'but if I'm going to be a doctor when I grow up I shall have to dissect things.'

Sure enough, when he cut it open he found the fish was

15

black inside, presumably from cement dust.

Because Gerry had so many other interests, he decided he would have to restrict his medical activities to five days a week. On Saturdays he was going to be an ornithologist, and on Sundays an organist!

His passionate interest in birds was reflected in the paintings he did at school, some of which I still have, framed and hanging in my sitting room. Typically, they depicted a bird of prey eating the bloody remains of a fish or some other creature. One picture of a sea eagle, painted when he was seven years old, appeared in an exhibition of arts and crafts in Holy Trinity Church. We lived in an ideal place for bird watching, with herons, oyster catchers, eider ducks and even the golden eagle to be seen in the area.

To help Gerry realise his ambition to be an organist, we bought a small organ on hire purchase, but the difficulty was finding someone who was prepared to teach him. It seemed he would have to learn the piano first, but piano lessons for him and Bram were discontinued after only a few weeks. It was difficult for me to take them into Dunoon for the lessons and neither of them liked the piano teacher much as she kept saying she much preferred teaching little girls! Gerry continued to play the organ his way, which he enjoyed, and we thought that perhaps one day he might get the chance to have organ lessons.

Ardentinny was a marvellous place for the children to grow up. The hotel stood right on the shore of the loch, with a grassy area leading down to the beach behind the hotel. The beach offered innumerable possibilities for games and exploration for three growing boys, of course. Gerry loved swimming, especially with a snorkel, and was always brave when it came to getting into cold water. He swam practically the whole year round.

Then there was fishing. When the mackerel were running, Gerry and the other two boys would go out in a boat and catch some for dinner. It was fascinating to see the water 'boiling' with the great teeming shoals of fish. Then was the time to go out on the loch and come in with a good catch.

The garden was a great place for birthday parties in fine weather. Photographs bring back memories of one such party held for Gerry's birthday — July 10th. It was a scorching hot afternoon and we had to fix a battered old sunshade to the table to keep the chocolate cake from melting. There was lots to eat, and fizzy lemonade to drink, and after tea the boys and their friends had only to run down the steps to the beach where they could play games or swim if they liked.

Barney and Nick the dog enjoyed outside parties too, for they usually got some titbits. One day an irate man came to the front door.

'Your pony is eating our picnic,' he almost shouted.

'Where are you having your picnic?' I asked.

It turned out that his family were lunching in our garden, so it was hardly surprising that Barney had joined them. I found him with their butter wrapper stuck to his nose. He loved having a picnic!

Barney made quite an impact on the village, for he had a habit of escaping from the garden and wandering round nosing into people's dustbins and turning them out all over the road. One day he did this trick in our own garden and I found him with the contents of two full bins spilled all over the place and Nick helping in the mess looking for interesting things.

Barney usually stood outside the window looking in when the guests were having their breakfast. We discovered he was getting titbits from them, so it was no surprise he peered in at them!

One day the boys had a great thrill. A helicopter landed in the front garden. The pilot and engineer had booked to stay at the hotel while they carried out work for the Forestry Commission. Their arrival was quite a hilarious event. When he saw the helicopter coming, Barney made a quick dash for the rhododendron bushes. Nick was in the garden too. Suddenly the wind from the rotors whisked Barney's plastic water bucket across the grass after the dog. Poor Nick, totally bewildered at being chased by this strange machine *and* a plastic bucket, also made a dash for the security of the thick bushes.

When the helicopter had landed, the boys rushed out, along with some guests who had been having dinner at the time. Barney and Nick peered round the bushes and gradually their curiosity got the better of them and they joined the crowd round the machine. The boys were thrilled to get a ride in the helicopter all round the village. Later Paul and Bram were able to go for a longer ride and help the pilot and engineer with their work. Gerry was disappointed not to be included with the older boys, but proud to have been up for a ride.

Among his other projects, Gerry spent hours designing houses for lizards and other small creatures to live in, as well as aquariums for different kinds of fish. Most of these designs got no further than the drawing book, but they gave him many hours of interest.

As well as the goldfish, Gerry liked to keep other fish, especially ones he had caught. One year a short holiday in England with his grandparents was made perfect because his grandmother took him to catch tiddlers in the park. He came home on the train with a large tin containing tiny fish: sticklebacks, redthroats and baby minnows. Shortly after his return I was changing the water for his treasured collection and decided to put them in the sink. Before I had returned them to their home I accidentally knocked the plug out and the tiddlers went away down the drain. I desperately tried to rescue them, even going as far as unscrewing the 'S' bend under the sink, but all to no avail. The little fish were all gone, down to the sea. I think I was more upset than Gerry who was quite forgiving.

Barney was quite an old pony when we got him and, sadly, he became ill. The vet diagnosed kidney trouble. After only two days Barney became too ill to stand. We called the vet again, but he was unable to come immediately. For about four hours I stayed with the dying pony in his field. The midges were very bad that evening, and his white coat was black with the horrible little insects crawling all over him and in his nose and eyes. I used up a can of fly-killer trying to keep them off him, but it was no use. I had to have a thin nylon scarf over my face to keep the midges off me. It was all quite horrible, as Barney lay dying, and I thought how awful it must be to see human beings dying covered with flies as happens in many poor countries.

Barney died before the vet arrived, and it was a relief when he was finally at peace. Gerry took Barney's death very philosophically, upset to have seen the little pony suffer so much, but knowing that he was at last away from his pain.

Not long after this we had another sad loss. Nick, in his mad boisterous way, had a habit of chasing after cars. He did it once too often one morning just before Easter 1972. He was hurt too badly to be saved and Trevor had to take him to the vet to have him put to sleep.

A short while before Nick's death he had mated with a lovely labrador bitch at a farm in Blairmore, some three miles down the road. Later on, when the pups were born, we went to choose one and ended up coming away with two — one each for Gerry and Bram. These two dogs, Glen and Rover, were to cause their own share of heartache in the months to come.

5. A TERRIBLE BLOW

Running a hotel meant a very full and busy life. We learned to welcome the winter, which gave us time to relax and have a normal home life. During the summer there was little natural home life for the boys as I was always so busy.

'Out you go,' was my constant command from the kitchen table where I stood or sat preparing food for the guests.

During the winter we were more relaxed. Often I would sit by the fire, with Bram and Gerry cuddled up beside me on the settee, and read to them. Our favourite books were the Narnia Chronicles by C.S. Lewis. Gerry's favourite was always *The Last Battle*, perhaps because in that story all the people we had been reading about in the seven books of the series went on to eternal life, leaving behind all the wars and unhappiness of the world. For two years we read and re-read the stories about the Narnia folk.

Christmas 1972 was coming and Gerry began to get headaches. The headaches got worse and he spent most days lying on the settee. He always felt sick and did not seem to be responding to the treatment he was having. By Christmas Day I was convinced he was dying. I accepted it — he had had a good remission, and I thanked God that Gerry had been with us for as long as he had.

During that Christmas Day I had an overwhelming feeling that it would be the last one we would spend together as a family; the last Christmas with Trevor, Paul, Bram, Gerry and me all together. I clung to every moment. I took lots of photographs (which didn't come out properly!) But the next day I realised how foolish I was. Where was my faith? I contacted all my Christian friends and asked them to pray for Gerry. Then I threw myself at the feet of Jesus and

20

asked Him for help.

A few days later, when the time for our visit to the clinic came, Gerry was already feeling better and was more himself. The spinal fluid test showed a definite improvement.

The doctor told me, 'He is responding to treatment at last.'

Or was it a miracle?

It was during that autumn and winter that I began to get very concerned about my husband. He had lost almost two stones in weight over the previous three years and had become very bad-tempered, particularly with the children. While overwork was partly to blame, another reason was that he just couldn't accept Gerry's illness. Trevor was often away, but when he was at home he would sometimes wake me up in the night to ask, 'When will he die?' It saddened me that, not sharing my faith in God, he wasn't able to accept the gift of Gerry's life, however short, and the joy it had brought us. Often he would talk about Gerry's 'hard luck in life'.

During the autumn before that fateful Christmas I became convinced that Trevor was heading for a nervous breakdown. Eventually, in November, he left his job and decided to devote all his time to the hotel. Perhaps it was because I was so worried about my husband at that time that I had not thought to ask my friends to pray for Gerry earlier. For some reason I did not think to ask for prayer for Trevor himself.

When he announced, after New Year, that he had decided to take a short break in Norway, I was pleased. Not only did I think it would do him good but, quite frankly, I was beginning to find life at the hotel very difficult with him always there. He seemed to have become extremely jealous and resented my attention being given to the guests, the hotel, or even the boys.

I took my husband to the ferry and wished him a good holiday. We arranged to pick him up the following week after a visit to the clinic. The week flew past, and I looked

forward to seeing a renewed husband the following
Tuesday.

Gerry and I duly turned up at the appointed time, but we
were disappointed not to see Trevor on the ferry, so we
went home. We expected to hear news that evening but
none came and I began to fear that something terrible had
happened. I realised that I had no address at which to
contact him. He had told me often that he had a friend who
knew Norway well and had recommended a holiday there. I
toyed with the idea of trying to contact this man. I looked for
Trevor's briefcase, thinking the address might be there. As I
searched I wondered if he really had gone to Norway.
Perhaps he had had a breakdown, and was wandering
somewhere — but where?

The more I thought about it, the more I realised how little I
knew of the Trevor of late. We had been so close for years,
but since we had had the hotel we hardly saw each other to
talk to. I reckoned that, if I found his briefcase, I would also
find the addresses of friends in England to whom he might
have gone.

When I eventually found the briefcase it was locked. I felt
bad about forcing the lock, but by then I was desperately
worried. When I opened it, I revealed a nightmare — so
common these days, but something I had never dreamed of.
Letters from a woman; photographs of Trevor with a strange
woman, on holiday it seemed.

I was totally numbed. So this explained all the strange,
and what I had thought unreasonable, feelings I had had
about my husband. He had been living the sort of double life
that makes a good story for a play on television. The sort of
story where the viewers laugh because the wife doesn't
know that she is sharing her husband with another woman.

The next week was terrible. I confided in my mother, and
in my friend the rector of our church. He advised pretending
to the boys that Trevor had gone for a fortnight and that I
had made a mistake. Paul was very suspicious, but Bram
and Gerry innocently went on living normally. By the

following week Paul had to be told, and the rector took on that job for me. At fourteen years old it was a terrible blow for Paul, but he took it manfully.

Two weeks later Trevor phoned us. He was in Newcastle, and could I collect him off the ferry at Dunoon at a certain time. He spoke casually, as though nothing had happened. I told him I knew where he had been. There was a silence, then I replaced the receiver.

It's hard to think clearly and objectively about the weeks after Trevor returned. I was so angry and hurt and lost; Trevor was so confused and, seemingly, now so hardened in his attitude to me and the children. There were faults on both sides, I suppose. Perhaps we had just taken on too much with the hotel and had not even noticed that we were drifting further and further apart. I don't know what the reasons were — but I do know that Trevor seemed to change into a totally different person from the loving husband and father I had known.

In the end, after much deliberation, Trevor decided to leave us. The morning after he told me of his decision, I went down early to make breakfast for Paul and Bram. I felt absolutely stupefied. What would we do? How would we manage?

Then I had the most unforgettable experience. As I went into the kitchen I saw Jesus there. He was standing in the middle of the kitchen with His arms outstretched towards me. His love enfolded me completely, and all my fears left me. I knew then that, whatever happened, I was safe in the arms of Jesus for ever and ever.

The day before Trevor had arranged to leave we told the children. Or rather, I told them. Bram and Gerry both cried. Gerry sobbed inconsolably for three hours. I had feared that the shock might be enough to kill him. I really believed that Trevor might change his mind when he saw how upset they were, but he didn't.

I took my husband to the ferry on the day he left. He spoke casually, implying that he would not be away for long. But by then I knew that the feelings I had had on Christmas Day were justified. Almost certainly we would never spend another Christmas together as a family. As I drove home I thought about the vision of Jesus I had had a few days earlier. I thanked God for giving me that assurance just at the time when I needed it most. I knew that He would take care of the family and that we were in His hands.

To my great relief, all three boys were wonderful. They seemed to think only of me during the sad days after Trevor left us.

'I'll look after you when you're old, Mum,' said Gerry.

What a joy it was to have him at that time, and to have the love and support of Paul and Bram. My mother and Trevor's mother were wonderful, and my father-in-law, never a demonstrative man, telephoned me to say, 'Look here, I'm the "old man" now. Don't hesitate to call on me for help, will you.'

Much to my relief, Gerry's health was not at all impaired by the trauma — another miracle, I believe. Our friends and staff rallied round us, and together we struggled through another busy season. I began to have some trouble with my heart though, and one day, to everyone's horror, I passed out in the kitchen. I was back on my feet within minutes, picking up the broken pieces of a basin in which I had been mixing a cake. My mother's heart was not very strong either; the doctor said it was 'wearing out'. I began to think that the hotel was becoming too much.

Questions flooded my mind. Should we give up the hotel? If so, where would we go, and how would we manage financially? But by now I was beginning to live by faith completely. I stopped worrying and surrendered myself to God and His will. I took even the smallest problem to our heavenly Father, so it was not hard to leave this matter with Him.

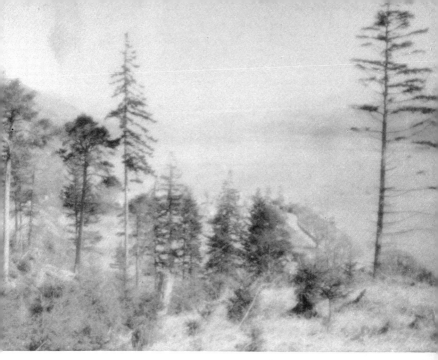

Loch Long with Ardentinny in the distant foreground

Gerry in Glen Finart

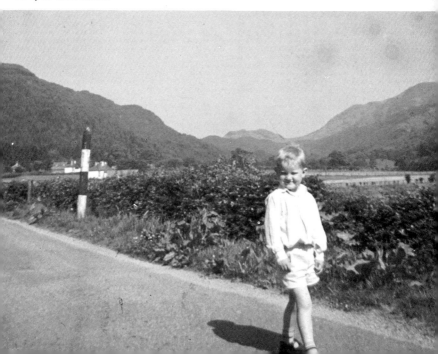

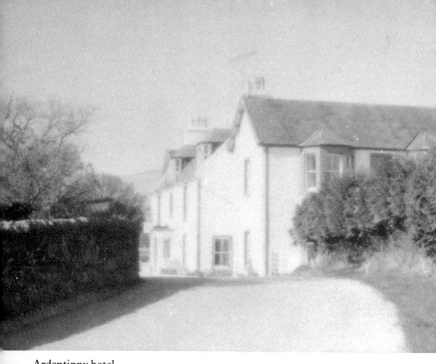

Ardentinny hotel

Gerry on Barney

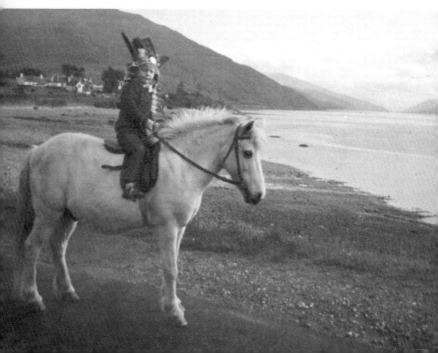

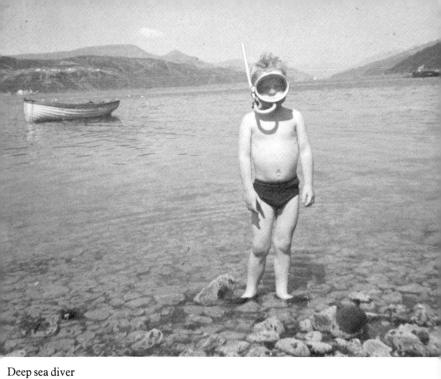

Deep sea diver

The three boys on the beach with Nick

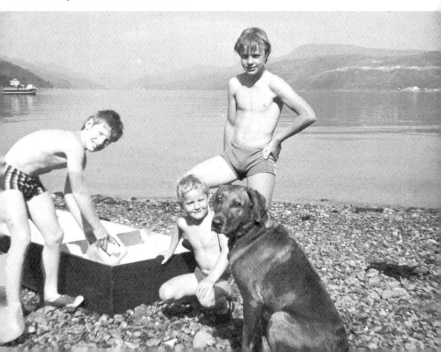

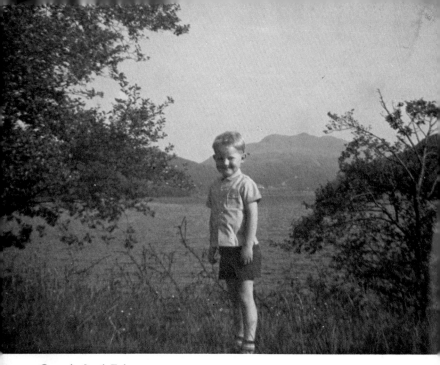

Gerry by Loch Eck

Ardentinny school

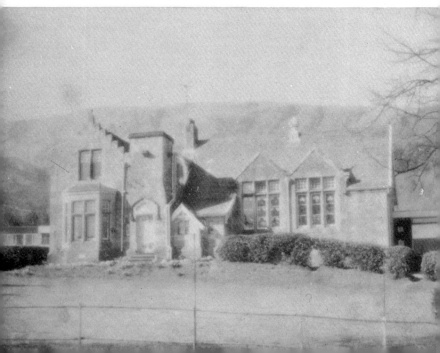

6. A KICK IN THE PANTS

In September 1973 I had the opportunity to attend a conference entitled 'The Charismatic Movement' on the Isle of Iona — the first conference of a religious nature I had ever been to.

What a week we had! We had a tremendous sense of the Holy Spirit's presence all the time, and everyone was lifted up to the heights. But we were warned by one of the speakers, 'Beware when you get home from here. Now you are on the crest of a wave, but Satan will give you a kick up the behind if you are not careful!'

I was soon to receive my 'kick'. My mother-in-law, who had come up to help my mother at the hotel while I was away, came to meet me from the steamer with Gerry. I could see at once that he was not well. Apparently he had been fretting for me. However, he did seem to perk up after I returned.

My mother-in-law went back to England, and life began to get easier in the hotel. We had closed for the season a few weeks early, because of my week in Iona, and now we just had the bar to run. What bliss it always was to close the hotel to residents. Of course, we valued the patronage of our guests, but after we closed we always felt free. We could run around and shout and scream if we wanted!

Gerry and Bram laid out their secondhand electric car set in the dining room, which made an ideal playroom in winter. Paul and Gerry were also very keen on war games. In fact, Paul and his friends had very serious games of the Battle of Waterloo. He and Gerry painted their little soldiers with great care, Gerry emulating his big brother by painting his plastic soldiers as painstakingly as Paul painted his lead ones. 'An investment' Paul proudly called his beautifully painted men. Another favourite game was 'Battleships', played on the dining-room carpet with rulers, dice and the large-scale plastic model ships the boys had made. Bram was never keen on war games — he was always the electrician who kept the car set going.

A few weeks after my Iona trip came the October holiday. Schoolchildren in Argyll get a week's holiday towards the end of October, the traditional potato-harvest holiday. It is a help to all those in the tourist trade. Tired parents who cannot get away in the summer months get the chance to go away for a short break with their families. The year before we had done some touring in England, and now we wanted to see a bit more of that country, especially old ruins and interesting places. We were all looking forward to our holiday — but it was not to be.

Gerry was still attending the clinic fortnightly, and a visit was due the day before we were to leave for our break. He had been troubled with slight headaches now and again, but had seemed much better after his off-colour spell a few weeks earlier. He was due for a spinal injection, which he hated. It meant all day in the day-bed area of the hospital. Only those who have had one know the agony of those terrible injections.

Gerry was always so brave about his injections. He loathed them, but he never made any fuss. He would curl himself up as the sister had shown him, tucking his head as far into his knees as it would go. It always made him so hot. We eventually persuaded the doctors to allow him to wear only his underpants, and not the towelling gown which made things worse and which used to imprint his flesh with marks of the cotton.

Red faced, with his golden hair clinging to his sweating face, Gerry would lie perfectly still for the fifteen or twenty minutes it sometimes took to get the anaesthetic in, wait for it to take effect, and then to find the elusive spot in his spine where the thick needle could go through to his spinal cord. Fluid would then be drawn off into a container for tests. Finally, a drug was injected into his spinal cord.

On this particular occasion, the doctor had to measure the pressure in Gerry's spine. Eventually the vital spot was found, the measure affixed, and the fluid allowed to find its level. It shot out of the needle and nearly hit the ceiling, well past anything the measure could record!

There was an awful silence. They say that ignorance is bliss, and I certainly did not realise how serious things were. But I sensed they were bad. Recovering himself, Gerry's doctor said that he must not be moved for a while as his spinal pressure was very high.

After the injection, he took me aside and explained that Gerry was very ill. It appeared that he had all the symptoms of a brain tumour. Any violent movement could cause the pressure in his spinal cord to touch his brain. I was quite numbed by it all. Gerry took the fact that he must lie still philosophically and seemed unconscious of the atmosphere of near-panic.

After about two hours resting on the treatment-room table, Gerry was wheeled up to a room in one of the wards. Exhausted, he fell asleep. I sat beside him praying for guidance. I felt very strongly that he should not be in hospital. I wondered if I was just being unreasonable or whether it was another of those intuitive feelings which I had come at last to respect.

The answer to my prayers came around six o'clock. Gerry opened his eyes and said, 'Take me home, Mum.'

'All right, darling, of course I will,' was my instant reply.

To the horror of the junior staff on duty, I dressed Gerry and carried him down to the car. The young doctor on duty unhesitatingly told me that my action could kill Gerry, as he was too ill to be moved.

Trusting as usual in the Lord, I drove carefully on the way home. Surely, I reasoned, it would be better for Gerry to die going home, happy and with me, than to die in a miserable state of mind in hospital. By the time we reached the half-way point on our journey home, Gerry was sleeping soundly on the back seat of the car.

I had phoned my mother from the hospital and she greeted me anxiously at the front door. Gerry was still asleep. Paul and Bram crowded round the car, Gerry woke up, and he promptly sat up and got out of the car.

'Careful, darling,' I called anxiously, but he did not heed.

He went straight into the dining room with his new electric car and started to play with it. I gently persuaded him that he should go to bed, and was relieved when he was sleeping peacefully in his own bed in his own room. I decided to sleep in a spare bed in the same room, just to be on the safe side.

The next day Gerry seemed fine. He wanted to play with the car set, and was not at all keen to rest. That evening at the hotel we had a meeting of our local preservation society of which I was the secretary. What a job I had concentrating on that meeting!

Later, I decided to telephone all my Christian friends again — including some I had met on Iona — and ask for prayer for Gerry. He was to need much prayer during the weeks to come.

7. CRISIS

On the Sunday following our hospital visit, Gerry seemed very ill indeed. All he wanted to do was lie on the settee in the lounge. I read to him, but he was not really interested. I prayed for strength to face whatever I had to face. I knew God was with us and that He would do what was best.

Sometime in the afternoon Gerry opened his eyes and said, 'Mummy, I feel so ill.' He closed his eyes and sighed.

I thought, 'This is IT.' I just gazed and gazed on his face, so beautiful as he lay there resting. How I loved him.

Again he opened his eyes and said, 'I feel so ill, Mummy.' He closed his eyes again, and I wondered how much longer he would keep on breathing.

There was a tap on the door and I crept across the room. It was my mother to say that a kind friend from the village had just brought Gerry a gift from the Harvest Festival at the church. I took the bunch of grapes and the jar of honey and returned to Gerry. He was lying there so peacefully. I put the things on the little table beside the settee.

Suddenly blue eyes were looking into mine with a smile. Gerry sat up.

'I think I'll have my tea,' he said.

'Oh God, how merciful you are,' I prayed in thanks. Gerry started on the grapes and was delighted with the honey; he had some in a sandwich for his tea! My mother's face lit up when I ran to the kitchen to say, 'Gerry wants some tea', though she had not known how near death he had seemed that afternoon.

How can one describe the relief and joy felt in a house when a sick loved-one recovers? Joy unbounded — words are so inadequate to express it. My mother-in-law was with us again, having been telephoned when the crisis occurred. She had arrived in time for Gerry's recovery. Tension released, we were all able to laugh again.

The next morning Gerry's doctor telephoned from Glasgow. He begged me to take Gerry back to hospital. He promised I could stay with him; that Gerry could take any toys he wanted; that we would have television. I think he would have promised the moon to get us into the hospital. After three quarters of an hour I reluctantly agreed to take Gerry back. I felt like a traitor in a way I couldn't understand.

As soon as Gerry was in hospital, he had a spinal injection and lots of tests. They were sure he had a brain tumour. Gerry himself did not seem overly worried, and ate and slept well. I found sleep nearly impossible. The nurses seemed to clatter up and down the corridor in exceptionally noisy shoes, and to stand outside our room for long conversations in the middle of the night. The heat was unbearable, and the night noises of the city nearly drove me mad.

One night I was reading a book to Gerry when I happened to look out of the window. The city of Glasgow, with all its lights, was spread out below. As I looked I noticed a tall office building right in the centre of the city. It's lighted windows formed a huge cross!

I have never seen this before or since, and I believe it was a special sign to remind me that our heavenly Father was still taking care of things. However, when I pointed the cross out to Gerry he didn't seem unduly interested. He just wanted me to keep on reading!

Life in the hospital was very different from when Gerry was first a patient. Now the children's hospital was in a new building. The modern wards had separate little rooms for the children whose mothers could stay with them, mum sleeping on a folding bed which was put away in the daytime. Each room had its own toilet and shower. There was a neat little kitchen on each ward, so if Gerry didn't like the food on the menu (mothers had a choice as well as the children), I could always boil him an egg. I could also make myself a welcome cup of tea or coffee whenever I wanted. Little things like that made life in the hospital more tolerable.

Television was also available, though the one portable set on the ward was usually in use by a twelve-year-old girl having intensive chemotherapy for leukemia. She was under a huge canopy which blew down a curtain of sterilized air to keep her free from infection. She was in hospital for a very long time, to die later that year after a great deal of trying and painful treatment. Also on the ward was a youngster suffering from acute diabetes. She was in a room of her own, and was thoroughly enjoying all the fuss she was getting, surrounded by presents and dressed in a pretty nightdress. She was very good about having to be on a special diet.

In a room near us was another little boy with leukemia. Like Gerry, he too had been in and out of hospital. In another room was a child who looked like an overgrown baby. The mother was being given a rest from caring for her child, who would never be anything more than a 'baby'. A good way to find out how blessed we are is to go into a hospital and see how others in this world are making out — often in far worse circumstances than ourselves.

Gerry's doctor had said that he would be able to tell me exactly how Gerry was on the Wednesday afternoon. He said that I would probably be asked to allow him to have radiotherapy — a thing I was very much against, for it would mean having it on his head.

I was already unpopular with the hospital authorities because not only had I twice since Gerry's illness taken him home against their wishes, but when he was admitted this time I had refused to sign a form which gives the hospital authorities the right to do whatever they feel is in the interests of the patient, regardless of parental consent.

I was very anxious about what the verdict would be on Wednesday, and I wanted Gerry to receive the reserved sacrament of Holy Communion. I telephoned a curate at the Anglican Cathedral Church of Saint Mary in Glasgow whom I had met on Iona. Unfortunately he was just leaving for London, but he advised me to telephone his superior, the provost of the cathedral.

When I heard the soft West Country accent of Mick Mansbridge on the telephone, I knew I would like him. I asked if Gerry could receive Holy Communion on Wednesday morning. Mick was to become a long-standing friend of the family. He is just the right sort of person to 'minister' to the sick, and the little service he held for us that day was exactly what we needed.

I accompanied Mick to the lift after the service and told him that I was to be informed that afternoon whether or not Gerry had a brain tumour. I told him that I expected them to want to give him radiotherapy and that I had decided to say 'No'. I said that I felt very strongly that it would be better for Gerry to die of that initial tumour than to go through all the terrible treatment and then, almost inevitably, develop secondary tumours and die anyway.

I told Mick that I knew, and Gerry knew, that there was a better life after this one, and that as a Christian it would be hypocritical to prolong Gerry's life here if it were likely to be a life of suffering.

'What would you do?' I asked.

Few people would have had the honesty to answer, as Mick did, 'I would do the same as you — not let them give him the radiotherapy.'

I was due to see the doctor in the afternoon, but before zero hour came the family arrived for a visit. Gerry seemed full of beans and was thrilled to see the boys and his grandmothers. How grateful I have always been for a mother and mother-in-law who are good friends and who are always there when needed. Had all been well, the three boys and I would have been away on holiday by now, but as it was Paul and Bram were making the most of the break at home. After all, we did live in such a lovely place that it wasn't necessary to go away from home to have a good time.

While Gerry and the family were still chatting the doctor came for me and we walked up the corridor to an empty lecture room. It seemed huge and dark, with high windows looking out across Glasgow. The doctor took his seat behind a table and motioned me to sit on the other side. I looked at him and prayed for strength to take whatever he had to say. As he began to speak I noticed for the first time that he was inclined to stutter.

'Well, er, Mrs Murton . . . I have to tell you . . .'

'Why didn't he hurry?' I thought.

'. . . it, er, really is quite extraordinary, but you see . . . there doesn't seem to be anything wrong with Gerald now.'

What was he saying? My mind couldn't quite grasp it.

He went on, 'You see, Gerald seemed to have all the symptoms of a brain tumour, but you know these things happen sometimes . . .'

I think he spoke for a bit longer, but I was not really listening. I was silently, in my heart, praising God our loving Father for letting Gerry stay with us for a while longer.

Gerry was able to come home from the hospital immediately, and how we rejoiced! Our family doctor, himself a Christian, came to see us.

'They sent me a report from the hospital the other day,' he said. 'They didn't think Gerry would live, but now look at him and at what they say. It's a miracle!'

8. TADPOLES AND TRAUMAS

Gerry was able to go back to school when the October holiday ended, and by the following spring he was full of vigour again.

Although he still attended the hospital clinic regularly, no one could have guessed that he had leukemia. Fortunately, Gerry himself never knew that there was anything seriously wrong with him. I remember on one occasion the boys were quibbling about sharing the same cup to drink from.

'Don't be fussy,' Gerry said, 'I haven't got a deadly disease.'

Dear child, I had thought at the time, little did he know.

But despite his illness Gerry continued to live a normal happy life. As he had grown older, his interest in birds, insects and the microscopic life of the pond had intensified and he was always busy with some project concerning the wild creatures that so fascinated him. He carefully saved up all his Christmas and birthday money and the fifty pence pieces I gave him whenever he had to have a big injection, and equipped himself with binoculars and a microscope.

Whenever I think of Gerry during that period, I see a boy with blue eyes and golden hair, jam-jar in one hand, fishing net in the other, ready to go off on an 'expedition' to find some more interesting creatures.

About a mile from where we lived was an old bomb hole which had become filled with water and oozy mud over the years. It was an ideal place for pondlife. Often his fishing net would consist of a length of wire and a piece of old net curtain — anything to catch those interesting specimens he loved! He kept diaries recording details of all the birds, insects and pondlife he found, and at home he had two 'ponds' — old sinks filled with water in which he kept the creatures he brought back from the bomb hole.

That April, when we had the outside of the hotel repainted, tragedy struck the inhabitants of the 'ponds'. The painter, seeking some water in which to clean his brushes, washed them in Gerry's sinks! I remember spending hours with Gerry trying to rescue the tiny tadpoles and other creatures with a strainer and putting them into clean water again. Those which were still encased in a little spawn seemed to be the ones which survived. Poor Gerry, so often things like that happened to him.

One day Gerry came running into the kitchen with an excited report of a strange creature he had found in his pond. It turned out to be the larva of a drone-fly, a maggot-like creature with a retractable tube which it uses for breathing by poking it up above the surface of the water. He was always so thrilled whenever he discovered a new creature he hadn't seen before.

In many ways, especially in the world of birds, Gerry taught me a great deal. I can now recognise many birds I did not notice before, and I find myself looking out for unusual insects which I can identify with the help of Gerry's numerous books on the subject.

The loss of the tadpoles was the least of our problems that spring. At Easter we had a fire in one of the bedrooms. Some newly-arrived guests had put their nine-year-old daughter up to bed on her own and, being small, the child had not been able to draw the curtains properly and had pulled them over an electric convector heater. At about nine o'clock, when I went upstairs to see if Gerry had finished his bath, I met a frightened little figure in a nightdress running downstairs.

'There's a fire in the bedroom,' she sobbed as she rushed past me.

I ran along the landing where the glow from the bedroom door was already intense. The sight was quite horrifying.

Flames — hundreds of little flames — were licking across the ceiling. The paintwork round the window was blazing furiously, as were the old shutters. I noticed that the window was jammed open about four inches where the new paint outside had caused it to stick. A stiff breeze blowing through the window fanned the flames.

I had automatically picked up the fire extinguisher from its position at the top of the stairs as I had run to the bedroom. I prayed hard as I squirted the jet from the extinguisher, first at the ceiling and then, as it quenched the flames, down to the floor. Surprisingly soon, the fire was out. The smoke was thick on the newly-painted landing. Then I noticed that everyone from the bar was in the doorway offering to help. For some reason nobody had thought to call the Fire Brigade!

To make certain the fire was out, I emptied another extinguisher all over the area. Then I telephoned the emergency operator and requested the Fire Brigade.

A few moments later a voice answered, 'Police Station.'

'I want the Fire Brigade, there's a fire in the hotel,' I said.

'Oh, they're out,' came the casual reply!

Fortunately, however, the relief Fire Brigade were able to come out and they arrived within half an hour to check that the fire was really out. Free pints all round were their reward for coming although, thankfully, they had no work to do.

The real tragedy occurred the next day. I was getting ready to go to the Good Friday service in Dunoon. Bram and a friend wanted to come with me and go to the swimming baths.

'You must take the dogs for a quick walk first,' I commanded a reluctant Bram, so the two boys ran off along the beach with the two labradors, Glen and Rover. Alas, the dogs were too quick for the boys. While they were examining the wreckage of a boat on the beach, the dogs ran away.

As they had previously killed sheep, I had to telephone

the local farmer on whose land I guessed they would be. An extensive search then began, a trail of dead sheep leading the men up the hill, high above the hotel. Bram's beloved dog, Rover, was shot. They could not find Glen, Gerry's dog.

Hours later I heard a bark at the back door. There was Glen, so pleased with himself and wagging his tail at me. It was awful. I knew he had just come from the killings; who could blame a dog? I got him in and bolted the back door. Then I telephoned the local gamekeeper who had been out for hours with the other men looking for the dogs. He came quickly, and I had to put Glen on his lead and take him out to the van. He too had to be shot. We later learned that it was a mistake to have two dogs in an area like ours because the pack instinct makes it more likely that they will worry sheep.

How was I to break the news to Gerry and Bram? Gerry had lost his first pet rabbit, killed by a dog when it had escaped and hopped down the road. To protect his feelings we had told him that the rabbit had run off to live in the wild. But Glen and Rover! The truth could not be withheld from the boys.

Bram was heartbroken at the news. When he loved, he really gave his whole heart. Gerry took it more calmly and seemed to be able to get his priorities right in a very adult fashion. Though seemingly so gay and light-hearted by nature, he was sometimes strangely wise and serious for a young boy. In addition, he was always so interested in birds and nature in general that I think his dog had occupied a smaller part of his life than was the case with Bram.

Nevertheless, we were all very sad to lose the dogs in such a tragic way, and ours seemed an abnormally quiet and empty household over the following weeks until we got used to being without them.

9. TIME TO MOVE ON

As it turned out, that was to be our last season in the hotel. Both my mother and I were finding it hard to cope with the tremendous amount of work and responsibility we had in running the business and bringing up the boys. Towards the end of the season, two unpleasant experiences with guests made us feel that we were indeed being pushed into getting rid of the hotel.

We had had a booking from a party of eleven miners from Yorkshire for a week's fishing in September, a period when we were always short-staffed since by then our student helpers had gone home. In the event only seven of the men could come, and when they arrived it was just as well. I don't know what they expected, but apparently it was very different from what our establishment could offer. Their first request, after 'More grub, lass', was 'Where's the lassies then?'

Having been a London policewoman before I married, I was used to handling difficult situations, but before the end of the week I had to tell one of the men to leave. Things had got beyond a joke when he expected to slap and tickle the proprietress while she was waiting at table! The men were also disturbing the other guests when they returned late at night, merry with drinking, from a neighbouring pub.

One night they were inadvertently locked out and I had to go downstairs in my dressing gown to let them in. I got chased upstairs for my trouble! I was really angry by this time, and had to ask them all to leave. When they had gone I began to wonder if this was one way in which the Lord was telling us to give up the hotel.

We had another nasty experience only a week later. A couple had booked in for the night; they arrived well before dinner and were shown to their room by a schoolgirl who helped us out at the weekends.

'I don't like them,' she said when she came back to the kitchen.

They did not come down for dinner at 7.30 p.m., and so I asked another of our helpers to go up and call the new arrivals. She too came down with the report that she did not like them. When they eventually did come down, the couple made themselves quite unpopular in the dining room where they dawdled over their meal, frustrating the waitresses who wanted to set up the tables for breakfast.

Next morning, when the couple were due to leave, the man looked at his bill and refused to pay the full price. He complained that their room was not very nice, the food hardly edible, and in fact became quite unpleasant and abusive. I was upset, but instead of bursting into tears, which was what I felt like doing, I managed to be angry in return. Nevertheless, they still refused to pay the full price and they drove off having, literally, had free drinks all the previous evening.

After they left I rang the local policeman. He pointed out that he could not really interfere in what was a civil case, but said he would come out anyway. Meantime he asked for a description of the couple's car and on the way over he met them on the road and stopped them. He examined the car in the hope of finding a fault, but it seemed to be in good order. He also found out that the man was employed as a chef in a big hotel on the east coast of Scotland. Having no cause to hinder them any longer, he came on to see me. I was very grateful for his support, and also for the fact that he verified the man's name and address with his employer — an action which would at least probably cause the man some embarrassment.

The boys were naturally upset by the events, and I could see Gerry was nearly in tears. We felt so helpless in these sorts of situations, especially not having a man about the place. I thanked God that it was the end of the season. With relief we closed the hotel part of the business. At last we could relax. The strain of the season, which seemed to get greater as the years went by, was over for another year.

Now that we were less busy, I had more time to think seriously about giving up the hotel. I began to feel very strongly that recent events were God's way of showing us that the time had come to move on. But where would we go? We did not want to leave Ardentinny because we all loved the village so much. Houses — particularly houses large enough to accommodate our family satisfactorily — were very difficult to come by, and recent oil developments had sent the price of any available property sky high.

There was hope that a Forestry Commission cottage up the road in Glen Finart might soon come on the market. It was next door to a dear friend of ours and, though small, had enough garden for my mother to have a residential caravan beside the house. Speculating, Mum and Gerry and I visited the Caravan Show in Glasgow one hospital day. Soon we were having ideas about the cottage, planning to have bedrooms made in the roof, and imagining what it would be like to live there. The house had not even been put up for offers, so goodness knows how long we expected to wait.

Then an old lady in the village died who had lived in a little house beside the school.

'This is it,' I thought. 'The Lord has taken the dear old soul away so we can have her house.'

At ninety-six years old she had had a good life and, happily, died without illness. She was just found dead in the living room as though she had fallen from her chair. We had all been very fond of her, and I felt sure she would not mind us having her home.

More planning and ideas followed. A caravan would still be needed, but at least the little house was bigger than the cottage up the glen and it was also much more convenient, being in the village proper. After the funeral I wrote to one of the old lady's daughters asking about the property. Our hopes were dashed however when she replied that she was hoping to keep the house for herself as she lived in a teacher's tied house and had no other home.

By this time we had advertised the hotel for sale. We had had a lot of interest, and the painful job of showing people round our home was in progress. The boys, like my mother and myself, felt a mixture of excitement and yet sadness at the prospect of leaving the hotel. We even toyed with the idea of letting the bar half and living in the rest as a house. Somehow that didn't seen right though. I just knew all would be well.

'Trust in God,' I tried to tell Mum.

'It's all right for you,' she answered, 'but I'm not so sure!'

We advertised for five weeks in the local paper for a house. All we were offered in reply were a two-bedroomed bungalow and a big old house needing a lot of renovation and too near the nuclear submarine base for our liking. Time was getting on and the hotel season would be starting at Easter. Prospective purchasers of the hotel were negotiating with solicitors, and we still had nowhere to go. Two friends offered temporary accommodation in their holiday cottages. I had faith that the Lord would look after us; He did, of course.

It was at about this time that Gerry developed a sore ear. The trouble came to a head one hospital day. We had to stop the car for a while as he was in terrible pain. Years earlier, just before we moved to Scotland, he had had an abscess in his ear. This seemed to be another.

By the time we got to the hospital the pain was dreadful. I asked that we sit in a room away from the other children because of Gerry's pain. If Gerry had not been so brave, had he screamed in pain instead of quietly moaning, he would have been dealt with more swiftly. As it was, he had to wait his turn to see the doctor.

When he eventually did see him, the doctor was appalled

and quickly called an ear, nose and throat specialist because the abscess had just burst in Gerry's ear. Fortunately the doctors were able to treat the ear, but it prevented him from swimming again that year — a great disappointment as he was very keen on swimming and wanted to earn another badge.

Soon after this ordeal a friend told me that Inverchapel Farm was for sale.

'That's not Ardentinny,' I thought ungratefully. Then I remembered that I had promised to let God lead us in whatever direction He chose, even if it meant leaving our beloved Ardentinny. I handed the whole matter over to Him once again.

10. INVERCHAPEL

I knew Inverchapel Farm slightly, having been there once. Although barely three miles from Ardentinny, over the hill, it is ten miles away by road. Still, I reasoned, that was not foo far to keep in contact with friends.

I went round to the farm that very afternoon. The owner confirmed that he and his wife were hoping to sell and that they were thinking in terms of fifteen thousand pounds. I asked whether I could bring the family the next day to view. The owner said we could view anytime, so off I went with the news.

'Oh, but it's not Ardentinny,' said all three boys.

Faces fell, especially Gerry's. The move would be hardest on him for he would have to change schools and leave most of his friends behind. Leaving his ponds, too, would be very difficult!

The following day our friends Mick Mansbridge, the provost of Saint Mary's cathedral, and his wife Margaret were coming to stay. As it was getting near Easter Mick was taking a short break to prepare himself for the busy time of Easter services ahead. It was good to see them, and I was grateful to have a man's opinion of the farm we were considering buying.

The day Mick was with us we inspected the water tank which was situated a few hundred yards up the hill. The big concrete tank looked enormous. The owner said it was no trouble to keep clear. All the same, we had had the experience of the Ardentinny water supply and knew that hill tanks can be a great trial.

Despite this drawback, the farm was really just what we

43

needed. In the farmhouse itself there was a large kitchen with an old Rayburn stove, a sitting room, two bedrooms and a huge old-fashioned bathroom downstairs. Upstairs there were another three bedrooms. The plan was that my mother could have the two downstairs rooms for a bedroom and sitting room, Paul and Bram could each have a bedroom, and Gerry and I could share the largest bedroom.

There were also a number of outbuildings including an old dairy, a washhouse, a tool-room, a byre and several barns. In fact it was simply ideal for us — much better than a poky little cottage where we would all be on top of one another.

In addition to the buildings, there were six and a half acres of field, hill, woodland and garden — all terribly neglected, but with enormous potential. Gerry began looking for places to make new ponds and a den, and each time I visited the farm I liked it more.

We started planning in earnest. The owners had decided to raise the price slightly, but we knew that what they were asking was a fair price for the time. If we wanted Inverchapel Farm we would have to pay the asking price. I contacted our solicitor immediately. Meanwhile, two parties were still interested in the hotel, and we were confident of a good sale. We took guests at Easter and, quite frankly, we were glad that it would be the last time. On 24th May 1974 we moved out of Ardentinny Hotel.

It was arranged that our furniture would be packed into the barn at Inverchapel, and we were to stay at one of the holiday cottages in Ardentinny for two weeks before the previous owners of the farm moved out.

God had his timing right. By the time we moved I felt so ill I couldn't imagine how I had ever managed to run the hotel at all. Perhaps things had just piled up on me of late for my heart was giving trouble again. The boys and I literally 'fell in a heap' in our temporary home. My mother went to stay with her good friend, Eileen, fairly near Inverchapel.

Fortunately, Gerry's new teacher knew his old one, so they were able to exchange notes about Gerry's hospital visits and other details about him. Another good thing was that Gerry knew one boy at his new school, the son of friends who were soon to move to England. Mark was able to introduce Gerry to the other children when we visited Rashfield school to see about him going there after we moved. He also bequeathed Rabbie, his pet rabbit, to Gerry who was very pleased with his new pet.

It was quite fun living in the little cottage for a couple of weeks and being just a 'mum' again after nearly six years running the hotel. I adapted surprisingly quickly. The boys found the place rather cramped, though it was a good lesson for them to make them appreciate living in roomy houses. Finally the big day arrived and we all moved into Inverchapel Farm.

Prospecting for suitable sites for his two new ponds was Gerry's chief occupation when we first moved to Inverchapel. He was determined to dig a pond for his two goldfish which would need clean water and a water lily. The other was to be a 'dirty' pond, full of slime and interesting creatures.

One day Gerry came rushing into the kitchen with another strange creature he had found. It was a dragonfly nymph, and was just as ugly in real life as the illustration in Gerry's nature book showed! He put it back where he had found it after having a good look at it. Finding such creatures was always a great thrill for Gerry.

There were so many good places to site a pond, so many little burns and drainage ditches to dam, that Gerry didn't get further than a few excavations here and there that first summer. An old plastic bucket housed the plants he intended to put at the edge of the natural pond when he had made it: a wild yellow iris, a meadowsweet and a kingcup. Meantime we stood the bucket in a safe place at the side of a little burn near the barn.

As it was such a wet summer that year the big project was to make a den in the roof of one of the barns. The boys were helped by their friends Emma and Sophie who were home for the school holidays at their parents' nearby cottage. An old shed had been pulled down at their house and the bits and pieces were carried over to our house on the roof of their car. Ancient timbers and doors, even old bed springs, were used to make a floor for the den. When it was finished, the den was a great success. No one knew it was there, so the youngsters could lie hidden away up in the barn roof and see and hear all that went on in the yard.

Bram spent some energetic days damming one of the bigger burns to make a swimming pool. A farmer friend gave him some black plastic which he used, held down with rocks, to line the pool. The end result was impressive. Gerry, always the bravest when it came to getting into cold water, christened the pool. It was just deep enough for him to get wet above his waist, and he even managed to swim a stroke or two. Sadly, the next day the pool was wrecked by vandals.

That summer the weather was so cold and wet that no one would have gone swimming much anyway. Plans to go to the beach at Ardentinny never materialised. It was more the weather to 'potter about' indoors and, in the case of the boys, play in the den.

It was marvellous to have all the barns and outhouses as well as several acres of land, and there was plenty of room for everyone to have their own projects. I had often dreamed of living in a place like Inverchapel Farm, and now at last that dream had come true.

11. NEW ADDITIONS

The year before we moved into Inverchapel Farm we had acquired a new member of the household. Having been without a dog for several months, since the tragic loss of Glen and Rover, we missed having one. Ever since Paul had been a baby we had had dogs, and I felt it was time we found another one. Bram was not keen. He couldn't bear the idea of replacing Glen and Rover, and he was also afraid he might lose another pet. The point was often debated, but no plans were laid.

One day I called on a friend who had recently retired as matron of the local geriatric hospital. There on her lap was the sweetest little bundle of white fluff in the form of Mack, her West Highland Terrier pup. He was adorable. I immediately wanted one like him. We had always had big dogs, but they were always big eaters and took up a lot of room in the car. Here was a sensible-sized creature who would fit into a small car like ours — and he would not cost much to feed.

'Yes,' said my friend in answer to my question, 'I think there is one of the litter still left.'

I went to the house where a young American girl showed me the last pup she had. He was tiny, smaller than Mack. With one ear flopped over and one pointed up, he was a sweet white bundle of fluff.

I bought him and took him home as a surprise.

'Daniel,' I thought. 'Daniel in the Lion's Den, for that is what you will be like when I get you home to those three big boys!' The pup shivered on my lap as I drove home — he really was minute.

My mother and the boys were in our cosy sitting room by the fire when I eventually got home. What a surprise when I went in with the puppy! Everyone loved him at first sight.

'What's his name?' they all seemed to ask at once.

Before I could reply, Paul said, 'Ludwig von Murton.'

'What?' I asked in amazement. 'I thought Dan would be all right.'

'No,' said Paul. 'Ludwig — after the mighty Beethoven. I chose the name for our next dog some time ago.'

Bram and Gerry naturally agreed with Paul who, after all, was so much more intelligent than poor old Mum!

The name 'Ludwig' for a tiny bundle of a dog seemed ridiculous then, and even now people look surprised when we call him. I don't think the great Beethoven would have been very flattered by our Ludwig's behaviour. He turned out to be the most difficult dog of all to housetrain. In fact, he would not go out at all in the cold and wet. He preferred the warmth and comfort of the house, with the result that the carpets had to be shampooed frequently during the months after we got him! But despite this handicap we all grew to love Ludwig dearly, and Bram developed a special affection for him.

With the purchase of Inverchapel Farm we inherited a number of other animals. These included numerous bantams and ducks and a rather temperamental pet sheep with a deformed foot known as 'Old Nick'. Old Nick had a habit of getting into the front garden and eating the vegetables we were trying to grow. He also used to get very bad-tempered if one did not produce titbits for him. One day, after he had nearly knocked my mother over because she did not have anything for him to eat, we decided that we would have to have him slaughtered.

Gerry was keen to raise ducklings, so he put two duck eggs under a broody bantam hen in the chicken shed. A few weeks later he was delighted to find that one of the eggs had hatched. For some reason he decided to call the little squeaking yellow bundle 'Whirligig' and we put him,

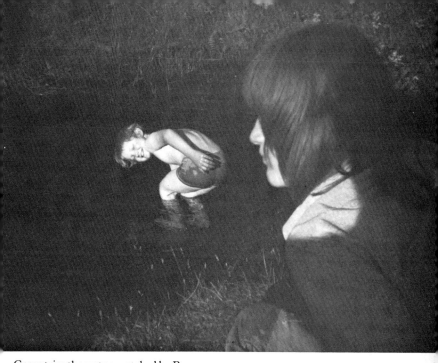

Gerry tries the water, watched by Bram

On holiday in 1974

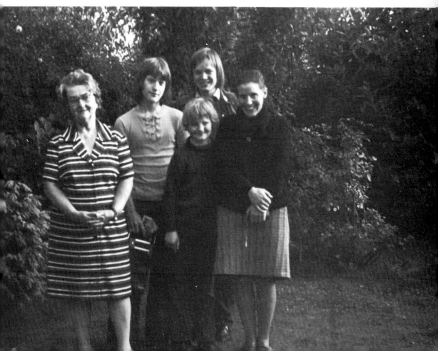

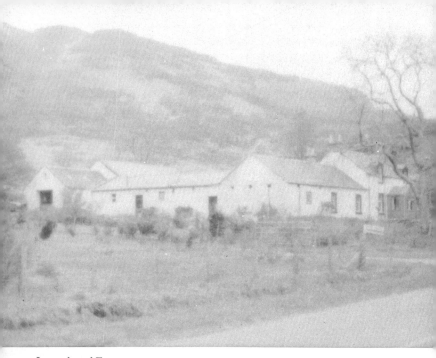

Inverchapel Farm

The three boys with Ludwig as a puppy

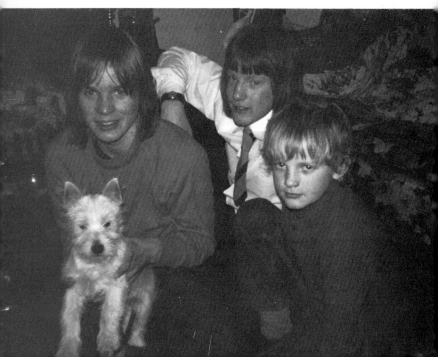

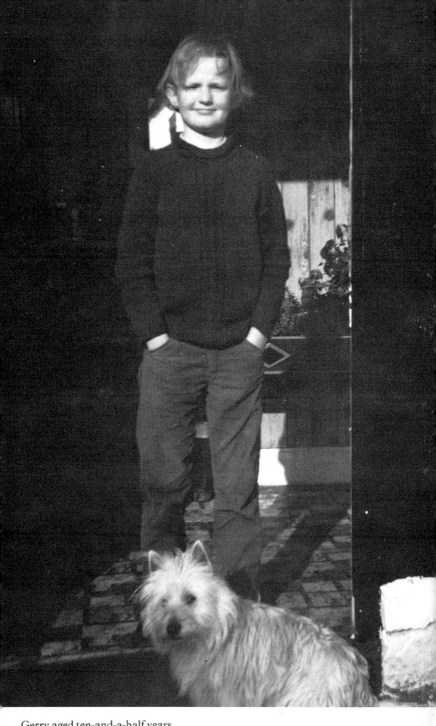

Gerry aged ten-and-a-half years

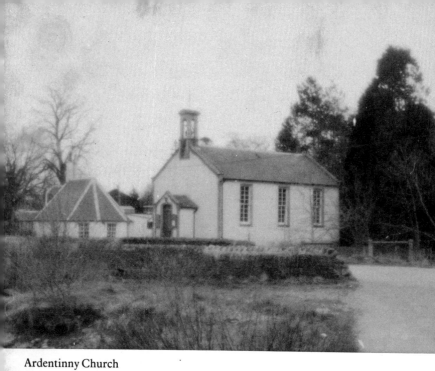

Ardentinny Church

Mary Kerr and Mary Murton in 1981

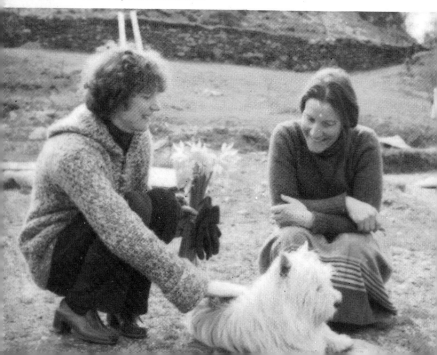

together with his proud foster mother, into a little run by themselves for safety.

As if we didn't have enough animals, what with Gerry's guinea pigs and rabbit too, the summer after we moved to Inverchapel we acquired a marmalade cat. He belonged to some American friends who were returning to the States and could not take him with them, so we offered Jasper a home.

The evening he arrived I took him, frightened as he was, from the arms of his owner who had brought him to our house. Ludwig was there and he jumped up at the cat. There was a terrific fight during which I was scratched across the nose. I have the scar still, and at the time the blood flowed freely everywhere.

After the commotion was over we realised that Jasper had disappeared. He had always been an 'outside' cat, but when he did not take the food we put out for him for several days we thought he had gone for good. We guessed that he might have tried to return to his old home, but that was eight miles away. Gradually, however, he began to take the food and milk we put out, although he was very shy at first and we hardly ever saw him.

In the event Jasper turned out to be a very useful member of the household. We were troubled with mice and rats at Inverchapel and, while I hate to kill any creature, there has to be some way of controlling vermin. Nature's method — a cat — seemed to be the answer. So we got a useful mouse-catcher and Jasper got a good home!

All that summer the cat was shy and nervous and the dog kept him in his place by chasing him every time they met. One day Ludwig chased Jasper across the garden. Jasper leapt into the laurel hedge and Ludwig carried on running through the hedge into the road. There was a terrible screech of brakes; Ludwig had run through the hedge straight into a car.

It was a terrible moment. The injured dog ran off, finally ending up at the house where my mother caught him.

Blood was trickling from his mouth. I prayed, 'Please God, don't let him be seriously hurt.' I knew Bram and Gerry would be heartbroken if they lost another animal.

My prayer was answered, and I am sure Mum had been praying too. Ludwig had only lost a couple of teeth, later found on the road by Bram. He was cut and shaken but, thank God, no real damage was done. We began to wish we had never had Jasper, what with Ludwig's scars and mine!

It was later that year that Jasper suddenly decided he was not an 'outside' cat any more. When we returned from holiday in October he was nowhere to be found. Apparently he had only taken his food for a few days, and then vanished. For two weeks he was missing. Gerry was sure he had gone to find his old home and that we would never see him again.

Then one day, without any fuss, in walked Jasper. He came right into the house, looked around as if to say 'Here I am then', and settled down as if he owned the place. From then on Jasper was the boss, not Ludwig. Though the dog still chased the cat, in a token sort of way, in the garden, his life was never the same again. Jasper even took to lying beside Ludwig on the hearthrug. But woe betide Ludwig if he should get too close — he was liable to come away with a bloody nose!

12. THE LONG WET SUMMER

That summer Paul decided to buy a student's travel pass with his savings. A friend of his had got a job in Germany, so Paul planned to go there first for a week; then the two of them intended to travel by train through Europe, ending up in the far north of Norway. Staying *en route* at my parents-in-law's house in Hertfordshire, Paul was driven in style to Dover by his 'Grandpa Ted'.

A few days after Paul left, my mother went to stay with my in-laws, together with her friend Eileen. The morning after Mum's arrival it was planned that the ladies would spend the day shopping and would have dinner ready for my father-in-law's return in the evening. He didn't arrive home for dinner, however, and there was no word from him during the evening.

They were just beginning to get really anxious when there was a knock at the front door. 'Nan Ted' opened it to reveal a policeman.

'Does your husband own an Aston Martin car?' he asked.

In the living room my mother's heart sank at the tone of the policeman's enquiry.

'I'm afraid I have to tell you that he has been involved in an accident,' continued the policeman.

Apparently the car had left the motorway, somersaulted down a bank, and he had been trapped inside. 'Grandpa Ted' was critically ill in the intensive care unit of a nearby hospital.

Bram, Gerry and I, still at home in Inverchapel, were numbed when we heard the news. We felt so helpless, and all we could do was simply wait and see what happened. I prayed that God would help the family and, if it were His will that my father-in-law should live, that he should not have brain damage as the doctors feared.

Their youngest son, the only one still in England, came into his own in handling his father's affairs and sympathetically assisting his mother in her bewildered grief. My mother and Eileen were also able to give 'Nan Ted' help and support.

As soon as Paul returned to England he telephoned me. I told him the sad news about the accident and that his grandfather was still unconscious after ten days in intensive care.

The next morning, Gerry was distressed to find the second of his baby guinea pigs dead. The litter had been born in the strained days of waiting for news, and the little mother was not being very good with her babies. That very evening his grandfather died.

'Oh Mum! Now we have no man in the family,' cried Gerry. It was hard to believe that the strong figure of Ted Murton was no longer on this earth.

The next day we discovered yet another sad thing had happened. Whirligig, the little duckling Gerry had hatched, was dead. I found him, battered to death, lying in the yard with a big bolt from an old telegraph pole lying across his poor bedraggled body. I couldn't hide my tears from Gerry, who was just going to school. He did not see the little body, but we were both too upset to do more than weep, and he could not go to school.

We discovered that a little boy from nearby had killed the duckling. He was renowned for being a violent child. Apparently he told his mother, 'I did shoot the duck — bang! bang!' As Gerry said, he didn't know any better.

How Satan was tormenting us! At every turn he was there, trying to take us away from the Lord. I had long ago learned that the more you try to live for Christ, the more Satan bedevils you.

Ted Murton's funeral was held on Paul's birthday and

mine — 2nd September. The following Monday Gerry cried at school; it was the beginning of a time of tearfulness for him. He really felt very upset that there was no longer a man in the family.

It was not essential for us to have a break in October any more, now that we did not have the hotel, but we decided that we would go away for a few days anyway. I felt that a holiday would do us all good. We decided on England again. Gerry was particularly keen on Roman remains and we planned to explore Hadrian's Wall and York, as well as visiting my mother-in-law in Hertfordshire and some other friends scattered around England. Paul was learning to drive, and the holiday would be an opportunity for him to have some valuable practice.

It was fortunate that Ludwig was small, for we had to take him with us. So off we set: Paul driving, me in the passenger seat and Gerry, Bram and Ludwig in the back seat. Ludwig was comfortably ensconced on a cushion to keep him happy for so many hours in the car!

Our first stop was the Roman wall and, in particular, Housesteads fort. Gerry was thrilled and so, for that matter, were the rest of us when we got to the site. The Romans called the fort *Vercovicium*, meaning 'hilly place', and it originally covered an area of around five acres. It was constructed in about A.D. 125 and would have housed as many as a thousand soldiers. While the fort is now in ruins, it is still possible to make out many of the features such as the remarkable latrine system and the pillars of the granaries which once supported a wooden floor allowing air to circulate underneath to keep the grain dry.

We spent a long time looking over the historic site. Gerry wanted to get a book on Hadrian and his army but, by the time he said so, we were already back in the car park — at least half a mile away from the shop on the site. I had to insist that he didn't go back because we were already late for our destination that evening, Reeth in Yorkshire.

We spent the next two days exploring the Yorkshire

dales. We had only passed through the area before, but now we had time to wander and we found it delightful.

Gerry had been particularly looking forward to going to York. He wanted to see the Roman remains of course, but he and the other two boys were also keen to visit the Railway Museum. They were so disappointed when we got there to find that, not only was the Railway Museum closed, but York Minster was closed as well because of a royal visit. We made the most of what we could do, however, walking round the quaint old streets and visiting the castle museum which the boys loved.

Ludwig was not very impressed with York. In fact he didn't like cities at all — all those feet and legs to get tangled up with! I usually ended up holding his lead outside some museum or other while the boys looked round inside.

Our next stop was Hertfordshire. Our feelings were mixed as we drove to my mother-in-law's house. We felt excited and yet sad. It had been difficult to believe 'Grandpa Ted' was gone before, but now, seeing his old home with him not there, the loss became very real to us.

It was good to spend some time with my mother-in-law and visit other relatives in the area, but soon we were off again — this time to visit old friends in Essex and Suffolk.

During the next few days we spent time in many of our old haunts. Happy memories flooded back; memories of us all together as a family, working hard, playing hard, making a home and a garden from a tumbledown house and a wilderness. Happy memories which were so precious and which outshone the unhappy ones.

The day we visited some very dear friends in a village where we had once lived, Paul was delighted to find that the son, whom he had not seen for three years, was home on leave from the army. He had been Paul's best friend at school. What a pleasant surprise that was, and what a time they had catching up on their news!

Many of our friends were surprised and delighted to see how well Gerry was looking. I think they expected a pale weakling after what they had heard about his illness. We visited a good friend, Gerry's godmother, on our trip to Essex. She was worthy of the name 'godmother'. Ever since she had learned of Gerry's illness she and her prayer group had been praying for him regularly. We valued her concern and prayer very much, as indeed we did that of all the people who had taken Gerry to their hearts and prayed for him (including a community of nuns as far afield as Australia!)

We stayed with some more friends in their converted inn in Suffolk. Their wood fire and huge inglenook reminded us again of happier days. The familiar Suffolk accent we heard in the local village was music to our ears. We explored the fens for the first time and discovered Ely: another beautiful cathedral; quaint old streets; echoes of history. We bought lots of vegetables in the area, finding them so much cheaper than at home.

The last night of our holiday we spent with Mark's family. (Mark was the boy who had introduced Gerry to the children at Rashfield school and who had given him Rabbie the rabbit.) Gerry was pleased to see his friend again and get re-acquainted. Poor Gerry, he had lost so many friends when he moved from Ardentinny that he had been delighted that Mark had been at the new school, even if only for a short time.

All too soon our enjoyable holiday was over. Mum was pleased to see us safely home and we all settled down for the winter, refreshed after our break.

13. MY ANGEL

Towards the end of November that year, the hospital became concerned that Gerry's blood count was too low, the lowest it had been since leukemia was first diagnosed. They said he should have a bone marrow test; he was very upset at the news, and became very depressed. The test proved positive and the doctor decided to start him on an intensive course of drugs. An immediate spinal injection was given. I later learned that at that time the doctor really thought that Gerry's case was hopeless.

When he got home Gerry went into a classic depression. He would not do anything other than sit on the old settee in the kitchen with his thumb in his mouth, staring into space. He couldn't go to school, he couldn't even write his name when I tried to get him to write to his grandmother. I prayed for guidance; it came.

'Take Gerry off the drugs and no more hospital,' a voice seemed to say.

Had I heard aright? Yes, it came again and again into my head. Perhaps it was imagination? I continued to pray; the 'voice' continued the message. The question was, had I enough faith to obey?

The following week Gerry was due for another visit to the hospital. Beforehand we went to the cathedral where he received the laying on of hands and the sacrament of Holy Communion. On the way to the hospital I decided to refuse any more treatment for Gerry. I had promised him that he would have no more spinal injections, and on that point I was quite certain.

Gerry's blood was tested and when we saw the doctor he

told us that there had been a dramatic improvement and that treatment could be restarted. Then, when I told him I did not want Gerry to have any more spinal injections, he looked despairingly at us. He asked if we would consider an injection in the hand. Gerry nodded; how weak I was to allow it. Poor child, it took three attempts of poking about under the skin of his already pin-pricked hand before the vein was located and the injection given. Another course of drugs was prescribed. I had begun to waver in my intention.

At home that night I excused myself weakly to Gerry about the drugs, and gave him his dose of the new medication. I tried to ignore the voice that kept nagging at me, 'No more drugs, no more hospital.' However, the next morning I felt strong. I prayed for strength to do what God wanted me to do. I did not give Gerry any more of his new drugs and he cheered up almost immediately. He went back to school, not too happily, but with me praying him through the day he managed. His parting words in the morning would be, 'Don't forget to keep praying that I won't cry or anything, Mum.'

Gerry didn't like school dinners and, not being a big eater at lunchtime anyway, he was happy to take a packed lunch. He always ate a good breakfast and had a dinner when he came home at night. It was good to see him getting back to normal.

I wrote to the doctor at the hospital to tell him I was not taking Gerry to the clinic for the time being. I told him that Gerry was not in the right state of mind for a visit and I did not want to upset him.

A week later our own doctor asked me to go and see him. He had had a letter from the hospital and he pointed out to me that they presumed I had guessed Gerry's case was hopeless. They were quite at a loss to understand why his blood count had fallen so low and why he had had a recurrence of leukemic cells. They could not suggest any treatment that would save him. I had not guessed the facts, but instinctively I had known that the hospital could do nothing more.

We continued to go regularly to St Mary's cathedral in Glasgow. There, in a little service held especially for us, Gerry received the laying on of hands and the reserved sacrament of Holy Communion. Despite his seemingly hopeless condition, Gerry was fine, well and happy, living normally again.

In fact he was so well that I thought there would be no harm in taking him to the hospital for a blood test. We went one week after the usual service in the cathedral. The test showed that the improvement in Gerry's blood had continued, despite him having had no treatment. The doctor was amazed.

'I think we've just made it this time,' he said quietly to me.

Christmas was approaching and the boys began to get excited. The Christmas season had lost some of its joy since Trevor had left. Nevertheless, we still loved the season with all the festivities and carol-singing to remind us of the Saviour's birth.

For the first time we had our own Christmas tree. The boys chose a very big one which took up so much room that we had to put the dining table in the barn! It was very beautiful, though, and we could always eat from the big table in the kitchen.

Gerry wanted to go to the midnight communion service on Christmas Eve in the church where we usually worshipped in Dunoon. It meant he would be up rather late but he enjoyed it, and we took the holy sacrament together at the altar with my mother. The service was late in starting, and Gerry was so sleepy that we had to leave before it was over.

That night I had to wait until late to make sure that all the boys were asleep before filling their stockings. Even Paul still liked to hang his up! As I crept around in the dark, trying to fill socks without making too much noise, I couldn't help thinking what a lot my husband had given up for his girlfriend.

Having been so late to bed, we were not very early

waking up on Christmas morning. The 'oohs' and 'ahs' of the excited boys as they opened the parcels in their stockings were so familiar. Usually I groaned and went back to sleep after the present-opening, but not this time.

Gerry was thrilled with some new toys, additions to his 'Action Man' collection, and a book of Bible stories by David Kossoff from his godmother.

'Look what I've got, Mum,' he shouted as he opened his parcels.

Then he and Bram ran downstairs to see what had been left under the tree. The parcels were poked about as the two boys tried to guess what was in them. Even Paul had a go to see what he was to get later when it was time to have the tree presents.

As I listened to their excited chatter, I thanked God that I had children, that I was blessed with such delights as the excitement of Christmas morning. Strangely enough it did not occur to me that we were unlikely to have Gerry with us for another Christmas. I could not really imagine Christmas Day without his happy face.

My mother's friend, Eileen, was with us for Christmas Day. After an enjoyable lunch of turkey and Christmas pudding we opened the presents round the tree. For some years Gerry had liked to dress up as Father Christmas. Wearing an old red dressing gown, a crepe paper hat and a cotton wool beard, he handed round the parcels. It was lovely to see the delight on loved-one's faces as they opened their presents. Truly it is more blessed to give than to receive.

Boxing Day was a complete disaster and it was entirely my fault. I had promised the hospital that I would take Gerry along for a check-up. We set off in a very un-Christmassy mood.

As usual, we went to the cathedral so that Gerry could receive the laying on of hands and the reserved sacrament before going to the hospital. Whilst waiting for Mick to come for the service, I had been looking at the bookstall at the back of the church. When he came in the side door, we both turned to go forward to the little chapel where the service would be held.

Gerry was sitting in a pew at the front of the church; the sunlight was pouring through the stained-glass windows in a shaft of coloured light which engulfed him. His golden hair glowed. I caught my breath, he looked so very beautiful — like an angel. 'Too beautiful to live here in this world,' I thought.

As Mick and Margaret were going out to lunch, and two other friends were also out, we had nowhere to go for lunch. Usually the bakers were open in Glasgow on Boxing Day, but not that year, so we had to be content with the canteen at the hospital. Gerry was very grumpy about that. He justifiably complained that I should not have taken him to hospital that day.

After a long wait in a full clinic, we were told that Gerry's blood was still normal. Why didn't I have the guts to trust God and leave hospital out of Gerry's life?

We just missed the ferry going home and had to wait an hour for the next.

Gerry said, 'I hope you're not going to mess up another Christmas like this one.'

At that moment I made up my mind for certain that there would be no more hospital.

Gerry went back to school, and life became normal for the first time in six years. No more drugs; no hospital visits. I asked Gerry how he felt without any tablets.

'Free, really free, Mum,' he said.

That was a good enough answer for me.

14. COMPLICATIONS

'Mistress Murton?' asked the man who had knocked at the back door. It was early February. Two men stood in the doorway. I vaguely recognised one from the hotel days.

'I am the Sheriff's Officer, and have come to serve this warrant on you.'

I gaped at him in amazement. I knew we still owed the previous owners the balance of the money for the property. Trevor still refused to sign the papers for the sale of the hotel, and they were threatening to take action to get their money. But this?

'I suppose you know what you are doing, Lord,' I prayed. 'I don't imagine you got us this lovely home just to have us kicked out, so I leave all this to you.'

I explained to the Sheriff's Officer my reasons for not having paid my debts. He was a very nice man, and he advised me to try and stall things a bit longer until the money was forthcoming.

'However, we will be back a week from today to value your property,' he said.

With those ominous words he and his silent companion, who I presumed was there as a witness to the serving of the warrant, departed.

It was all quite a shock, but the outcome was that my husband was persuaded to sign the appropriate papers after I agreed to let him have the piece of land I had retained from the sale and one or two other items. The money we owed was paid by the following week, so the Sheriff's Officer did not return.

Gerry still seemed to be keeping well and was happier

than he had been for some time. There was no more bursting into tears at school, although he had started to worry about going to the grammar school. He had another two years to go at Rashfield school, but was becoming concerned that he could not seem to do the school work he had found easy at Ardentinny school. I believe his brain had been damaged by all the spinal injections and drug treatment he had received.

I thought of Gerry's prayer for guidance years before, and I wondered whether he would ever achieve his ambition of becoming a doctor. Gerry knew God, and he trusted in His goodness and guidance.

That February everyone seemed to have flu and many of the children at Gerry's school were off sick. Inevitably Gerry caught the infection. I called the doctor in who gave Gerry something to ease the symptoms. The infection settled on his chest, which often happened. However, within a few days he seemed much better and was full of beans again except for a persistent cough which I thought would soon clear up. I sent him back to school the following Monday.

When he came home that afternoon after school he was quite cross with me. He told me that the other children with flu had been off school for two weeks while he was only off for one. I had to remind him that he had already missed a lot of schooling so he had to catch up.

On the Thursday Gerry's cough was too bad for him to go to school. On the Friday he woke up with pains all over him. He was still coughing and I had to go to the doctor's surgery for cough mixture for him.

The doctor's wife is a good friend of mine and, while her husband made up the medicine, we talked in her kitchen.

'You know, I think this is it,' I said. 'I think this may be the beginning of the end for Gerry.'

'Don't be silly,' she replied, 'it's only flu.'

But in my heart I knew that it was so.

15. DYING, WE LIVE

Gerry's cough gradually became worse, and by the Saturday afternoon he was having the most awful pain in his middle when he coughed. I called the doctor in who said the pain was from his spleen and liver. Apparently these organs had virtually given up working.

The doctor was sympathetic with my wish that Gerry should not go into hospital. As a Christian he shared my belief that this is but a transitory life to help us prepare for the life to come. I think he agreed with my view that we should not try to prolong life artificially when all hope is gone.

Pain killers kept the pain bearable for Gerry, and he was content with the diagnosis I gave him — that he had a touch of pleurisy. During the next few days he actually seemed quite well. He was up and dressed, and playing with his 'Action Man' on the lounge floor each day. I made sure he had his pain-killing tablets on time. However, by the next week they were obviously not strong enough. He was given something stronger. The doctor left an injection in case it was needed and he was not available. In that event the district nurse would be able to give it.

During this period I was reading the book *Dying, We Live* which I had bought from the cathedral bookstall. Gerry, seeing the cover picture showing prisoners lined up in front of a firing squad, had said, 'Why have you bought another of those horrible Nazi books, Mum?'

I had explained that books like that show us how people overcame the evil of Hitler's regime.

For me that book will always be a manual for life. In the letters from people sentenced to death for their opposition to Hitler, I found words of comfort and hope. Most of them had endured terrible hardship or torture before, eventually, being killed for their beliefs. Whatever I was suffering, they had suffered more. I thanked God that I had the knowledge and comfort of His presence to help me endure whatever was to come.

Gerry was happy only when I was near. He wanted me to embroider new badges for 'Action Man' — some of the new uniforms did not have such nice realistic badges as the ones Gerry had had some years before. He spent ages packing all his 'Action Man' things into boxes; one box for boots, another for guns, and so on. The whole time Gerry seemed to be packing up all his favourite toys to be 'put away'.

On the Wednesday morning I was in the kitchen, just through a curtain from the lounge where Gerry was playing. Suddenly he screamed — a terrible scream. I ran to him. He was standing in front of the chair where he had been sitting, his face screwed up in pain. He clung to me, sobbing; then he sat down.

We could hear my mother telephoning the doctor. Gerry was always very brave, so we knew the pain must have been excruciating to make him scream like that.

'Mum,' Gerry said, 'when Nan comes in I want you both to pray with me, to ask God not to let me have a pain like that again. I don't think I could bear it.'

My mother came in and we told her of the need to pray. She and I knelt by the chair where Gerry sat.

'Dear Father in heaven,' I prayed, 'please don't let Gerry have another pain like that. We ask in Jesus' name, Amen.'

'We had better pray again,' said Gerry.

'But darling, we've prayed once,' I said.

'You know what Jesus said about the woman and the unjust judge; we've got to keep nagging.'

So we repeated our prayer, and Gerry never had any more pain!

Our doctor arrived and brought a different medicine which was easier to take. The sun came out, and I remembered (or perhaps the Good Lord reminded me) that I had some film left in my camera from the holiday.

'Come on, Gerry, the sun is shining — let me take your photo at the front door, darling.'

I have a picture of a very fine young man, standing in the doorway in the winter sunshine. At the age of ten and a half he looks very mature, not a little boy at all.

Most of the next day Gerry stayed in bed and I read to him. He came downstairs to see television for a while, but there was nothing very good on. He missed 'The Goodies' now that their series was over. What a lot of pleasure they had given him, and indeed all of us, that winter. The sense of humour in their programme had appealed to us, maybe because we are a bit mad too!

The following day Gerry decided not to get up until he felt better. He still felt quite poorly, and was content to lie and listen to me reading to him.

The doctor called round that evening. I asked him if he had any idea how long Gerry would last. My mother-in-law was due up for her annual visit the following day, and I knew she would not want to leave again unless there was an idea of when she would have to be back with us. The doctor shook his head.

'You know what these things are like,' he said. 'It could be six weeks, could be two months. One just can't tell.'

That weekend a dear friend who is a priest and his wife were coming to visit us. Hamish Cook was filling in on Sunday at the church in Dunoon as the rector had recently left. When I learned that they were coming I telephoned and asked for Gerry to be given the reserved sacrament of Holy Communion on the Saturday.

When Hamish and his wife arrived I took them upstairs to join Gerry for the little service. He was quite sleepy by this time. My mother was with us, and we all knelt beside the bed. Hamish wore his ordinary clothes — frills were irrelevant at a time like this.

I was kneeling right beside Gerry, and Hamish, who was

at the foot of the bed, could not reach to give him the Body of Christ. So I took it from Hamish and gave it to Gerry, putting the bread into his mouth. Then I held the cup to his lips, and he drank the Blood of Christ. So simple, but so important.

A little while later my mother-in-law arrived. She was shocked to see Gerry so weak, but relieved that he was not in pain and looked so peaceful. He looked quite beautiful and he seemed to have grown up in the last few days. He was, as in the photograph I have, quite a young man.

As I sat beside Gerry's bed while he slept, he would occasionally open his eyes to ask the time or just to make sure I was there. I prayed he would not have to suffer the ghastly death that seemed inevitable. I had seen a close friend suffering that horrible slow cancer death. I wished it could be me lying there and not my beloved boy. The miracle of no pain continued. Gerry knew God would answer his prayer. Gerry knew God.

While Gerry slept I continued to read my book of the sufferings of those almost forgotten people in Nazi Germany. Dietrich Bonhoeffer is well known now, but many were famous neither before nor after their terrible deaths. What faith many of them had — faith that was to be rewarded in an uplifting of their spirits to the heights only those who know God through His Son Jesus Christ can know.

The words I was reading seemed so appropriate to our situation:

'He [God] cannot let us be tried beyond our strength, but will see to it that the trial comes to such an end that we can bear it . . .'

I had read the same message when Trevor was leaving us, although then I had turned up a page in my Bible at random. God truly speaks to us through His Word.

The Lord was preparing me, for as I read on I came across these words:

'Even the loss of a most beloved one does not rob us of happiness. After a short period of trial we shall be reunited with our loved ones in the Glory of God, and He will wipe away all our tears.'

16. 'I'VE TASTED BLOOD'

The next day, Sunday March 2nd 1975, Gerry woke at about 8.30. He had had a good night, but soon after waking his nose began to bleed. The blood was bright red and flowed so freely that everything was bloodied within a short time. Eventually I managed to stem the flow, and I laid him down gently with his head back slightly. He was very pale and upset and I tried to reassure him that his nose bleed had been because he was so weak.

A little while later he called out, 'Quick Mum, I'm going to be sick.'

My mother was there at the time and ran to fetch some towels. Luckily I was able to catch the blood he brought up in a towel, so he did not see the frightening extent of it.

'Is this a haemorrhage?' I asked myself. I had no experience of such things, but common sense told me it must be. Soon after, another bout of sickness followed. Gerry blamed me for stopping his nose bleed.

'It was better to have a nose bleed than this,' he said. 'Let's pray that God won't let me be sick like that again.'

Silently I prayed, 'Don't let him down, God. Please.'

Out loud I prayed for Gerry, 'Please, Lord, don't let Gerry be sick like that again. We ask this in Jesus' name, Amen.'

Gerry was not sick again.

Once more at peace, he sank back on the pillows.

'That's the second time I've tasted blood today, Mum.'

'Yes, darling, you were sick before, and you had that nose bleed,' I said.

'No, Mum. I had the *wine*.' Gerry had a tone of reproach in his voice as he looked at me. He obviously thought I

68

should have known. He did not seem to realise that a night had passed since he had taken the bread and wine, the Body and Blood of Christ.

I wondered at such a young person understanding the significance of the holy sacrament. I did not realise then that to Gerry the wine really *was* blood. He was being truthful, not clever, when he told me he had tasted blood.

The time had come for the service on the radio. I had been listening for the past two weeks to a series of three talks by a Roman Catholic priest. I asked Mum to bring the radio upstairs so that Gerry and I could listen to the service together. The theme of the talk was 'Let yourself float on the love of God' — just the sort of advice we needed. I was to continue repeating those words to Gerry for as long as he lived.

For the first time Gerry did not want anything to eat. He only wanted orange juice. 'Squeezed orange,' he said, so his grandmother squeezed the juice from fresh oranges. He had to drink from an old-fashioned china invalid's cup as I did not want to sit him up after all the sickness. He was, even then, quite amused at drinking out of a 'teapot'.

The doctor had promised to look in that afternoon, but strangely he called in the morning after church instead. He was amazed to find a peacefully dying child — no long weeks of suffering, no heartbreaking weeks of pain and despair. Gerry was going home to his Lord quicker and more smoothly than anyone had thought possible.

Gerry dozed a lot as the precious minutes crept into hours. I continued to sit by his bed. Now and again he would wake up, open his eyes, and say of the quilt on his bed, 'Take that thing off, I'm hot', and I would throw it off for a minute or two.

'Will he die like this, in my arms?' I thought at one time as he lay there so peacefully, his head on my shoulder. Then he became too heavy and I started to get cramp, so I put my head on the pillow beside him instead.

I wanted time to stop, to be with Gerry forever. Yet I did

not want him to suffer. When he woke I would say, 'Go to sleep, darling, you will feel better when you wake up.'

Twice Gerry tried to tell me something, but in my anxiety to hear what he said I couldn't catch his words.

'What did you say?' I asked.

'Oh never mind, I'll tell you later,' he said.

I have often wondered how long I will have to wait to hear what it was Gerry wanted to tell me. To me 'later' will mean many years, to him perhaps just an instant.

A few moments later it happened. I became conscious of a change in Gerry's breathing. The doctor, who had stayed with us when he realised the end was very near, went quickly from the room. I later learned that he was overcome with emotion and had gone outside where his tears would not be seen.

At the same moment I became conscious that the family were coming upstairs. Later they told me that they all felt a compulsion to come up to the bedroom at that very moment. My mother came and knelt beside me at Gerry's bed, my mother-in-law beside her. Paul was in the doorway, Bram just outside.

People had spoken of a 'death rattle', which I was dreading to hear, but thankfully there was nothing like that. After a few moments Gerry breathed deeply and then sighed; just one long sigh — an outpouring of breath, the breath of life. The boy I loved so much, my darling Gerry, had gone from us.

'It is finished,' I said and I threw my arms round him, thanking God for giving Gerry such a wonderfully peaceful death.

I remember thinking then, 'God is good; trust in Him and He won't let you down. But you have to give yourself to Him completely — no half measures. It's like marriage, only the love is greater than human love can ever be. It is a complete and utter sacrifice of oneself to Jesus. Through Him God will give you strength, He will give you peace. He will give you the morning star.'

So that was it, nothing frightening about death after all. I had never been with anyone who was dying before, but now I would welcome the opportunity to sit with a person rather than let them die alone.

We gathered in the lounge a little later where our doctor led us in prayer. It was all so calm. Death always comes as a shock, even if it is expected, but I knew that for Gerry it was a new beginning. I had sensed, as I sat beside his bed, that the Lord had greater work for him elsewhere. Gerry's work here was over. 'Mission complete,' Gerry would have said.

He went a long way away when he died, and I was glad. I did not want him to be bound to me or to this planet in any way; I wanted God's will for Gerry, and that seemed to be freedom.

After the undertaker had been I went up to the bedroom. Gerry's body was so strangely still and cold. His lovely golden hair still curled around his ears; what a beautiful child he was.

I turned to my Bible and opened it. I read, 'He will tend his flock like a shepherd and gather them together with his arm; he will carry the lambs in his bosom . . .'

The Word of God gave me great comfort.

17. A JOYOUS OCCASION

The dog did not like the coffin they put Gerry in. Poor little Ludwig, he and the cat had been very upset that day when Gerry had screamed. They had rushed into the room and hardly left us since. Up in the bedroom Ludwig had lain on the rug most of the time Gerry was in bed. Now, with Gerry gone and that nasty white box on his bed, Ludwig still lay there — so sad, not understanding.

On the Wednesday after Gerry died his funeral took place. Six years previously I had sat in Ardentinny church for the first time. Then I had choked back the tears as I had imagined what his funeral would be like. I had planned to have him cremated and his ashes sprinkled at Kilmory, Loch Sween, a beautiful place on the west coast of Scotland which Gerry had loved.

Then, just a few months before Gerry's death I had attended the funeral in a nearby village of a young girl who had died of cancer. I had wondered at that time whether the next funeral would be Gerry's, and if so how I would feel.

Now that the day had arrived, it was different from anything I had been able to imagine. For me, Gerry's funeral turned out to be one of the happier occasions in my life. For one thing I was able to rejoice that Gerry had lived to know God through His Son Jesus Christ. And I thanked God that in the end his death had been so peaceful and free of suffering.

The little church beside the loch at Ardentinny was filled to capacity with friends and neighbours when we arrived. Everyone was there, it seemed. There were Gerry's teacher and some friends from Rashfield school, along with the teacher and the whole of Ardentinny school except for the youngest ones. Many of our ex-staff members were also there and lots of other friends who had given us their help and support after Trevor left and to whom we owed so much. It was wonderful to feel the love of so many dear people as we entered the church ready for the funeral.

Paul and Bram were both still very upset and felt sure they would not be able to keep their composure during the service. On my advice they prayed for strength and, in the event, the church looked so lovely and the love of all the people so filled it, that their prayers were answered.

Flowers decked the church and Gerry's white coffin was covered with little posies from people's gardens. Spring had given us a few precious blooms and, together with the mass of flowers from the Dunoon florists, the scene was glorious. As we were ushered to the front of the church we saw that eyes were downcast and many people were crying, their faces smudged with tears.

It was a magnificent service. Mick Mansbridge took the funeral, assisted by the minister of Ardentinny church, and he gave the message of salvation to all present. He told them how Gerry knew God and that he was now with God. I sang 'The Lord's my Shepherd' and 'Just as I am without one plea . . . O Lamb of God I come' with all my heart and voice.

When the service was over we followed the coffin out into the sunshine. I found myself shaking hands with people and kissing them. I was filled with love for every person there, a special God-given love.

I saw Eddie, Gerry's best friend, standing sobbing. I went up to him and put my arms round him.

'Don't cry, Eddie, Gerry is happy now with Jesus,' I said.

His face brightened and I later heard that he told his mother, 'If Gerry's mum is happy, I will be too.'

People were crying, and laughing too. The message given at the funeral had touched many hearts, and I later learned that some of those present had been made to think very deeply about God by the experience.

We had arranged to have Gerry's body cremated, so that meant going by ferry to Gourock after the funeral. Our party consisted of the hearse and four car-loads of people. When we got to the crematorium the hearse and our own car with Paul, Bram and myself inside arrived safely at the entrance. No one else was in sight. We waited and waited but there was still no sign of anyone. The attendants, who were all dressed in the usual black with sombre faces to match, wrung their hands in despair. They looked so agitated, poor souls, that I wanted to laugh. I remember thinking how amused Gerry would have been by the incident!

Eventually the car containing my mother, mother-in-law, Eileen and another friend appeared, slowly crawling up the steep narrow driveway. Apparently it had broken down at the bottom of the hill and the two other cars were behind. Luckily Eddie's father, an excellent car mechanic, had been able to get the car going again. It turned out that the clutch had failed.

At the crematorium more friends met us, those who had not been able to make it across to Ardentinny. They were able to share in the little service held in the chapel. Again, the flowers were lovely. I was able to give some to a friend to distribute to sick people in Glasgow. Mick and Margaret also took some for sick folk they knew.

My mother had the bright idea of not leaving the remaining flowers at the crematorium to die, but taking them home instead. So we filled the boots of two cars and distributed the flowers to local old people's homes where they delighted the residents and lasted for quite a long time.

Gerry's ashes were buried at the Cathedral Church of Saint Mary the Virgin in Glasgow in a simple ceremony which took place two weeks later. My mother-in-law stayed with us long enough to attend the service, and several ladies from the cathedral Bible class asked if they could join us too. Again, Mick Mansbridge conducted the service, this time assisted by my friend the curate whom I had met on Iona.

For the burial service we all stood beside the wooden crucifix outside the cathedral. Though surrounded by family and friends, I felt strangely alone. I cast a hesitant glance at the terribly small casket which held all that remained of Gerry's mortal body. I hastily looked away again. The curate, noticing my glance, came and stood beside me comfortingly. I fixed my eyes on the purple primulas at my feet.

Suddenly, Gerry was there beside me. I glanced to my right — there was his golden head bowed beside me!

'Imagination,' I thought. No, he was still there. Yet it was more of a sense of his presence than a vision. I knew he was with me, and I was reassured.

The sense of Gerry's presence faded, and I was filled with peace. The words of Jesus came to me, and I again rejoiced.

'My peace I give unto you,
the peace which the world cannot give.'

AFTERWARDS

Looking back on Gerry's death, now six years in the past, I still find myself thanking God for the way in which it happened. Since then I have seen other people suffer so much from cancer in one form or another. At times the words of a hospital doctor echo in my head, 'He will die in agony, with tumours all over his body.' I have seen that happen to a very dear friend of mine and I continually thank God that Gerry was spared all the suffering, the long and terrible agony, which is all too common these days.

During the years since Gerry died I have found two new and very fulfilling interests in my life. I have started fostering and arranging holidays for deprived children, and I have also become deeply involved in the healing ministry of Christ's Church.

I began the work with children the summer after Gerry died. With the other boys nearly grown up, and Gerry gone, I felt that I had a lot of time and love to spare for needy children. I also had plenty of toys lying around which would only gather dust if they had no one to play with them!

The first two children to come for a holiday came from a very poor area of Glasgow. Since then one of the original pair has returned for a holiday each year. He has really become one of the family. I soon found myself *organising* holidays as well as providing them, asking people to take one or more deprived children from inner city areas into their homes for a week or two during the summer.

My involvement with children was extended when I became an approved foster mother. After having several short-stay children, I had two sisters for a period of two years. They were aged six and nine when they came to live with me, and they eventually left to go back to live with their mother who had remarried. They still keep in touch, and are always sure of a place in my heart.

Now I have a sixteen-year-old foster daughter who has been with me for some time, as well as my holiday children, and I am sometimes reminded of the comment in the Old Testament about the woman without a husband having more children than the woman with a husband!

Talking of husbands, one of my greatest joys is that Paul and Bram now have a very friendly relationship with their father. The boys go out to stay with him in Norway for holidays, and Trevor and the woman he lives with (we are not divorced) are very generous to my hard-up student sons. Also, Trevor and I have a friendly correspondence and I know that if we meet again there will be no bitter feelings.

Bram knows God now, and another thrill for me was when my mother came to a new and much deeper commitment to God after receiving the laying on of hands for her arthritis at a Catholic Day of Renewal. She was seventy-three years of age! I had the joy of hearing her stand up in church and tell all the people what God had done for her.

It was really through Gerry's illness that I became involved in the healing ministry of the Church. Many times during his illness Gerry experienced recovery after the doctors had considered his case to be virtually hopeless. These recoveries had followed times of concentrated prayer for Gerry and in some cases the laying on of hands and the reserved sacrament of Holy Communion. I believe that these were all ways through which God's healing grace was able to pour into Gerry.

At the end he died peacefully and with remarkably little suffering, and I believe that this was in a sense 'healing' too. After all, death was a new beginning, it was the pain and suffering that we were all praying would be alleviated.

I had often talked about healing with a friend of mine, Eric Fisher, an Anglican priest whom I had met on the Isle of Iona. He himself is what some would call a 'healer', although such people prefer simply to be recognised as channels through which God's healing power is made available to the sick and needy.

Eric was particularly interested in the miracles we believed we had experienced in Gerry's life and death. It was he who told me that Gerry had indeed tasted blood at that last communion service. I had thought that the saints of old were the only ones to taste the Blood of Christ, but now I know that there are saints in our day who do so. What a way to die, so close to Jesus!

But although I had seen healing miracles take place in my own son's life, nevertheless I was still rather sceptical of so-called 'healing services'. I had once attended one of the weekly healing services on Iona and seen people go forward to the altar to receive the laying on of hands. A disabled boy in a wheelchair had gone forward and afterwards I had seen him in the grounds trying to walk. I felt angry, for the boy was not really walking but just taking a few hesitant steps and I thought then that people had no right to give him false hope.

However, the autumn after Gerry died I had an experience which changed my opinion. I was staying with some friends in England who are what I would call 'violent' Christians, a term I fondly use to describe some of my more charismatic brothers and sisters! While I was with them they planned to attend a renewal meeting at a local church and, as it was to include a healing service, I decided I might as well go along and seek relief from the severe migraines I had been suffering from for several years.

When we got to the church I immediately felt at home. The uninhibited singing, laughing and praising God in a huge church packed with worshippers of all denominations seemed to be a glimpse of something I had always wanted to be a part of.

After a sermon on the second coming of Christ, the moment came for those who were seeking healing to go forward. There were several priests and ministers taking part in the service and they all made themselves available at the front of the church, ready to give the laying on of hands to anyone who needed it. Suddenly there were crowds going forward, and I was amongst them. I had read of such things happening and wondered what it would be like to share in such an experience.

Then I saw what I had not really believed did happen. People were dropping down on the floor like toy soldiers. They weren't crumpling up, as in a faint, but just lying down as if invisible hands were guiding their bodies gently to the floor in a prostrate position. One man beside me began to go backwards. There wasn't room for him so he remained propped up between me and the end of the pew!

I went forward and I remember that as the minister laid his hands on my head he spoke to me as if he knew all about me. I had a wonderful feeling, as if I were going up through the roof. I have never had a migraine since, and that is a real miracle. I used to have days when I could not move for the pain despite the strongest tablets available from my doctor.

Soon after this I witnessed other healing miracles. My friend Eric came to visit us for a few days and was able to help some sick friends of mine, some suffering from physical, others from psychological problems. One friend was healed of claustrophobia. She had been unable to go into big shops or indeed into any large building unless she stayed near the door. This had been going on for some years. She came to our house where Eric talked to her and then laid his hands on her head and prayed for her.

She told me later that immediately afterwards she had been able to go into a supermarket and right to the back of the shop where she had never been able to venture before. The same day she took the ferry to Gourock and went into the big department stores there. When she got home she triumphantly told her husband that she had been cured of a fear that had made her life wretched.

Another friend, the young mother of two children, had been very ill and leukemia was suspected. She was prayed for and received the laying on of hands. The next week we rejoiced with her to hear that the specialist had decided that after all she had pernicious anaemia and that she was already well on the road to recovery.

I began to think more deeply about the commands Jesus had given to his twelve disciples.

'Preach the gospel,' He had said. But then He had added, 'Heal the sick.'

Surely, I reasoned, the second instruction is as important as the first one, and yet so often Christians tend to ignore it. But now I was witnessing with my own eyes how this command to 'heal the sick' was being obeyed by His disciples in our churches today.

I was to experience, personally, another healing miracle in my own life. I had been suffering for over a year from severe backache caused, according to the X-rays, by a degenerate disc combined with a slight touch of arthritis. I was fitted with a surgical corset which was a most uncomfortable thing, but at least it eased the pain when driving. The pain had begun to make me very bad-tempered. My poor little foster children; I was becoming a very crotchety Aunt Mary!

It dawned on me one day, when I was going through a particularly bad patch of pain and immobility, that I was letting the pain prevent me from doing God's work properly. If I could not be happy and cheerful, then I was not shining like a candle in the dark. In fact, I was very much a spluttering candle!

Some time before I had been given a tape recording by Father Francis MacNutt, a Roman Catholic priest whose book *Healing* is one of the best-known on the subject. I decided to look out the tape which was on the subject of 'The Healing Power of the Holy Spirit'. Then I phoned a friend of mine, the Baptist minister in Dunoon, whose Bible study and prayer group was due to meet the following evening. I asked him if they would all pray for the healing of my back at the meeting.

The next night I put the children to bed extra early, telling them the reason. Then I put on the tape by Father MacNutt and lay down on my bed. As I listened to his voice, I tried to imagine my many friends praying at the church. I saw their faces; I loved them. Then I imagined myself opening out like a flower in the morning sun. I was opening myself to the Holy Spirit of God. At some stage I must have turned the tape over though I don't remember when.

When Father MacNutt had finished speaking I began to pray for all the people I knew of who were sick. I prayed especially for a little boy I knew of who had cancer. I did not know Neil personally, but he was the grandson of a friend of a friend.

As I prayed I felt very strongly that God wanted me to visit Neil's family.

'I can't, Lord, I don't know them,' I protested. But the voice continued and in the end I said 'O.K., Lord, I'll go tomorrow.' I also had the strong feeling that God was asking me to start a healing prayer group in Dunoon.

Excited at the prospect of getting a healing group going, and rather overawed at the prospect of calling on people I did not know, I jumped up from the bed. I had been up for a few moments before I realised that I had got up from the bed unaided and that I was standing upright with no pain. I bent forward — still no pain. I danced round and round the room; then I ran downstairs to tell my mother that I had been healed. What a wonderful feeling it was to be able to move around again without any pain!

The next day I visited Neil's family. It turned out that someone at the hospital in Glasgow had recommended to Neil's mother that she should get in touch with me! Neil, just six years old, was a very sick child when I first saw him. I spoke to his mother and his grandmother about my own experiences, and I think I was able to help them. A very deep bond of friendship was to form between us over the months to come.

A few days after my first visit I took a big box of Gerry's precious 'Action Man' things for Neil to play with. However, he did not need to be amused for long. A few more days, and the Lord took Neil to that 'exciting' place where Gerry had gone.

On other occasions I have felt compelled to tell someone Gerry's story, and it has always proved helpful to the hearer.

As well as the experiences of healing in my own life I have also been a channel for God's healing power. A man with lung cancer had had a relapse after a seemingly successful operation. He had visited Eric Fisher on an earlier occasion, but was not able to get down to England to see him again.

At his wife's request I visited them and we spoke on the telephone to Eric. Eric prayed over the phone and I laid my hands on the sick man and repeated his words. Nothing very much happened at first, but then the man felt a tingling sensation starting in his toes, and the pain gradually began to ease. In fact, the man died a few weeks later but that does not mean that the prayers were to no avail. On the contrary, he died more swiftly than expected and with less suffering. As in Gerry's case, I had seen that prayer can help a person to die in a more peaceful way.

I often think how much I owe to Gerry and his faith in God which was an example to us all. I think of how he would speak of heaven as being 'a much nicer place' than here, and I realise that but for his life and death I probably would not be involved in many of the things which now fill my life. Through Gerry I gained glimpses of God's grace of which I previously had no knowledge, and now my joy and fulfilment in life is serving Him.

The Bethesda Fellowship of Healing meets once a month in Dunoon. We have a long list of people needing prayer. Clergy and lay people of all denominations are involved, including Roman Catholics, Episcopalians, Baptists and

Church of Scotland members.

So it goes on, each of us trying to shine in our little corner of the world. If we all keep lighting other people's candles, what a wonderful glow there will be — a world lit up with the love of Jesus!